The HIGH FIBER COOKBOOK

DIA

by Mabel

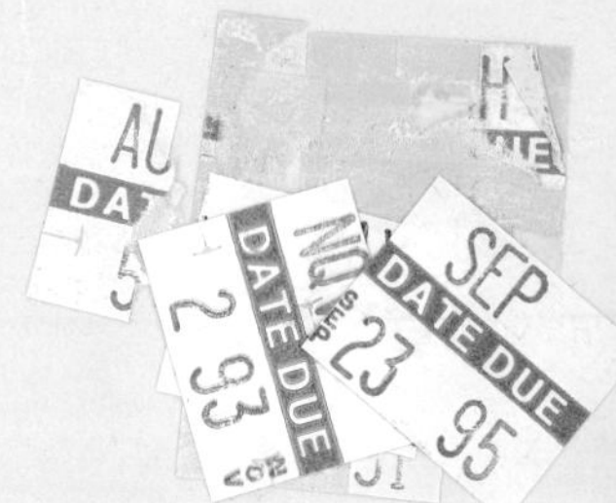

To Frances Nielsen, who taught me so much of what I know about cooking, the only person I know who cooks to relax when she is tired. The many hours we have spent talking about and practicing cooking have been among the best in my life.

Perigee Books
are published by
The Putnam Publishing Group
200 Madison Avenue
New York, NY 10016

Published simultaneously in Canada by
General Publishing Co. Limited, Toronto

The food exchange lists used in this book are the basis of a meal planning system designed by a committee of the American Diabetes Association, Inc. and the American Dietetic Association. While designed primarily for people with diabetes and others who must follow special diets, the exchange lists are based on principles of good nutrition and apply to everyone. The lists are copyrighted by the American Diabetes Association, Inc. and the American Dietetic Association and are used with their permission.

Designed by Helen L. Granger/Levavi & Levavi

Library of Congress Cataloging-in-Publication Data

Cavaiani, Mabel.
The high fiber cookbook for diabetics.

Includes index.
1. Diabetes—Diet therapy—Recipes. 2. High-fiber diet—Recipes. I. Title. [DNLM: 1. Cellulose—popular works. 2. Cookery. 3. Diabetic Diet—popular works. WK 819 C376h]
RC622.C37 1987 641.5′6314 86-25134
ISBN 0-399-51335-3

Printed in the United States of America
1 2 3 4 5 6 7 8 9 10

CONTENTS

	Acknowledgments	4
	Introduction	5
	Foreword by Dr. Joseph Crockett	9
1	Diabetes	11
2	Fiber in the Diabetic Diet	16
3	Food Exchanges	22
4	Planning Menus	41
5	Ingredients	46
6	Soups	53
7	Entrées	66
8	Vegetables	103
9	Salads	119
10	Yeast Breads	136
11	Hot Breads	149
12	Cakes	160
13	Cookies	180
14	Pies and Puddings	190
	Index	207

ACKNOWLEDGMENTS

I would like to thank the following persons for their encouragement and professional help in developing and writing this book. Without their interest and support I probably would never have written it.

Dr. Susan Urbatsch, of the Medical Clinic, West Union, Iowa, my family doctor, whose help and encouragement taught me there is life after diabetes.

Muriel Urbashich, R.D., Director of the dietary department of South Chicago Community Hospital, Chicago, Illinois, and her staff. Their generous cooperation and expertise have been a real help to me.

Mary Klicka, M.S., R.D., Chief; Patricia Prell, M.S., R.D.; and Jessie McNutt, R.D., The Ration Design and Evaluation Branch, U.S. Army Natick Research and Development Center, Natick, Mass. They have been so generous with their help when I had questions which only they could answer, and their expertise is acknowledged by everyone who has had contact with them and their department.

Mabel Frances Gunsallus, M.S., R.D., Miami, Florida, a friend of mine for many years with whom I have spent hours discussing this book and its contents as well as every other book I have written.

Edith Robinson, M.S., R.D., Decatur, Georgia, who first encouraged me to write books that she knew would be helpful to patients and to other dietitians.

Frances Lee, M.S., R.D., Dietary Consultant of Kerens, Texas, formerly head of the Experimental Kitchen at the U.S. Army Natick Laboratories, who is a friend in need when I am having trouble with recipes or any other problems connected with my writing . . . or my life.

Eva Burrack, Food Service Supervisor at the Lutheran Nursing Home and Gernand Retirement center, Strawberry Point, Iowa, and her dietary staff, who cheerfully tasted and discussed many of the recipes tested while I was working on this book.

Donna Beckstrom, Vice President of Golden West Medical Nutrition Center, Newport Beach, California, who is always encouraging anyone who needs to do so to use low-calorie recipes to improve their health.

Vera and Aulden Wilson, Wadena, Iowa, who tested recipes and listened to my problems while I was writing this and other books.

Garrieth (Butch), Jan and Johnathan Franks, our neighbors, who are always helpful and who make our lives here in Wadena much more interesting and enjoyable. Their help and friendship are a constant joy to Chuck and me.

And last, but certainly not least, my husband, Chuck Cavaiani, and my sister Shirley Sniffin. Their patience and support while I was writing this book have made it possible for me to be free to finish it.

I would also like to thank the following organizations for background information, resource material and nutritive information used in this book.

The American Diabetes Association, Inc.
The American Dietetic Association
The American Heart Association
Iowa State University Extension Service
U.S. Department of Agriculture
Iowa Affiliate of the American Diabetes Association, Inc.
Nutrient Data Branch, Human Nutrition Information Service, U.S. Department of Agriculture

INTRODUCTION

I probably sound like Pollyanna, but I honestly believe that people who follow their diabetic diet are, except for their diabetes, often healthier than those who live on junk food and don't get the proper amount of all of the necessary nutrients. I've always heard "You are what you eat," and it seems apparent that more and more people are beginning to realize the truth of this statement.

I frequently hear someone say to a diabetic "How well you look" in a surprised tone of voice. This always intrigues me, because I know that same person who is admiring the clear skin and evident vitality of the person with diabetes would probably look much better if they followed the basic diabetic diet. The diabetic diet, which includes lots of fruits and vegetables, a moderate amount of meat, fish, poultry and dairy products and a minimum amount of sugar, fat and alcohol, is the same diet our ancestors followed for thousands of years. In fact, the latest government guidelines for a healthy diet, which follow, are the same general guidelines which diabetics follow every day.

1. Eat a variety of foods.
2. Maintain a desirable weight.
3. Avoid too much fat, saturated fat and cholesterol.

4. Eat foods which are adequate in starch and fiber.
5. Avoid too much sugar.
6. Avoid too much sodium.
7. If you drink alcoholic beverages, do so in moderation.

These guidelines, which have been established for *everyone,* reinforce my conviction that families that include a diabetic would do well to follow a general diabetic diet, adding only those desserts and other indulgences that they feel they can handle after they have eaten the basic diet.

Exercise is very important to diabetics, and most follow a regular exercise routine depending upon their age and athletic abilities. My own exercise regime consists mostly of brisk walks and riding an exercise bicycle, but more athletic diabetics engage in even the most strenuous exercises, including marathons and long-distance bicycle races. This is something family members can also join to their own benefit.

Many people are concerned about their weight these days and as a registered dietitian I get many requests for help with weight reduction. I always recommend a basic 1200 calorie diabetic diet for weight reduction. It is well balanced, provides adequate nutrition and will certainly help anyone lose weight without starvation.

I have tried in this book to provide diabetics and their families with sane, sensible advice about diet, along with recipes that I think will be suitable for the whole family. I have not used a great many sugar substitutes because I honestly am not all that happy with the taste of most sugar substitutes, except of course for Equal (aspartame), and in most cases I have made the sugar substitute optional. There are a few recipes, such as the cranberry muffins, which require the addition of a sugar substitute, but I have tried to keep these recipes to a minimum. If you like the taste of sugar substitute and your taste buds react better to a sweeter taste, you can add more sugar substitute to the recipes without changing their food exchanges.

You will notice that in this book I frequently refer to the low-cholesterol diet. I have two reasons for this. One very important reason is that seventy-five percent of diabetics die of arteriosclerosis or a related disease which is aggravated by a high cholesterol count, so I think that all diabetics should be careful of their cholesterol count. The other reason is that my husband, Chuck, had a high cholesterol count, and after he had been on a strict low-cholesterol diet for some time, he brought his count down to low normal, so I am convinced that a low-cholesterol diet is very sensible and effective. I think that almost everyone should follow a low-cholesterol diet, particularly anyone who is diabetic . . . we certainly do at our home and I hope that you do also.

A diet that is high in fiber is also very helpful for diabetics, so I have included recipes with a good fiber content. At the moment there is so much discussion of fiber that everyone has heard about the benefits of a high fiber diet. I hope you have heeded all of the good advice, which is sensible for anyone who is trying to control blood sugar as well as for anyone who is trying to prevent constipation.

Most of these recipes are suitable for your family, and I'm sure they will like them. I'm not particularly happy about most "diabetic" or "dietetic" foods. Frequently they cost much more than it would cost to prepare them at home and unless you read the label very carefully, you can't be sure they are really good for your diabetic diet. They often contain sorbitol or fructose, which do raise your blood sugar, or something else not helpful for your diet.

Nutritive analysis of foods and recipes is very important to diabetics so they can determine how many food exchanges are included in their food. I have analyzed recipes for food exchanges based upon the 1986 revision of food exchanges made by the American Diabetes and the American Dietetic Associations' joint committee. Nutritive information included with recipes is based upon information in the following U.S. Government publications:

Nutritive Values of Foods in Common Units, Agricultural Handbook 456, U.S. Department of Agriculture, Washington, D.C., (783-3238) Superintendent of Documents, U.S. Printing Office, 1975.

Nutritive Value of Foods, Home and Garden Bulletin 72, U.S. Department of Agriculture, Washington, D.C., Superintendent of Documents, U.S. Printing Office.

Composition of Foods, Raw, Processed and Prepared, Agriculture Handbook No. 8, U.S. Department of Agriculture, Washington, D.C., Superintendent of Documents, U.S. Printing Office, 1963 and as many of the current revisions as are available at this time.

Preparing two different menus for one family—one for the diabetic and one for the rest of the family—has never appealed to me. Basically, a diabetic should be able to eat almost anything, except desserts and sweetened foods, that the rest of the family enjoys, and the rest of the family should be able to eat and enjoy all of the foods prepared for the diabetic. I don't believe in way-out recipes for diabetics. I think they should be able to enjoy foods prepared from items which are available in their favorite stores, with the addition of the occasional sugar substitutes and foods sweetened commercially with sugar substitutes (such as gelatin and soft drinks) and therefore I have included basic recipes with information which I hope will help you analyze your own recipes so you can use those also.

I don't want to give the impression that I think we are lucky to be diabetic, because we aren't. Diabetes isn't a fun disease. It is a very serious matter and I follow my diet, take my medication and exercise with one eye on the glucometer like everyone else. But it is a disease that can be controlled, and we need to give it everything we have to keep it that way. A diabetic diet can be dull and uninteresting or well balanced, tasty and appealing, and it only takes a little more effort to achieve that goal. I know I have appreciated all of the help that I have received from others in the past few years and I hope this book and its recipes and advice will help make your life and the lives of your family a little healthier and happier. If I have accomplished that, I will feel it has been worthwhile.

Mabel Cavaiani, R.D.
Wadena, Iowa

FOREWORD

by Dr. Joseph Crockett

Mrs. Cavaiani, a diabetic and a registered dietitian, is well aware of the needs and limitations of persons with diabetes. Because she is aware of those needs, she has collected and developed a collection of very palatable recipes for diabetics. She has also included other information which she feels will be of great help to diabetics. Her chapters on diabetes and the importance of fiber in the diabetic diet should prove especially interesting for diabetics and non-diabetics alike.

A regular and well-regulated diet is very important to diabetics. In fact, many diabetics can control their diabetes with diet and without any medication. A successful diet should allow the diabetic to continue to eat familiar foods. Anyone who is placed on a diet which includes a lot of unfamiliar foods is inclined to forget that diet and eat what they like. Because she wants diabetics to follow their diets, Mrs. Cavaiani has adjusted and included foods which are familiar to most diabetics and foods which are available in stores across the country. She has also attempted to bring a variety of interesting foods into the sometimes restrictive diabetic diet.

Most people who are cooking for themselves or others will find that these recipes are attractive for nondiabetics too. Therefore they will no longer need to prepare a separate menu for the diabetic but can prepare one acceptable menu to be enjoyed by the entire family.

Diabetes is characterized by a disturbance of metabolism and vascular changes. With diabetes mellitus there is typically a deficiency of insulin activity, altered fat and protein metabolism and a speed-up of fatty deposits in the blood vessels. Treatment aims to keep blood sugar as close to normal as possible, which requires maintaining a good balance between insulin, diet and exercise. Consultation with your physician will determine whether you need insulin or oral medication or whether you can control your diabetes with diet and exercise.

Research indicates that a good intake of dietary fiber and a diet high in complex carbohydrates will help control blood sugar, and a diet low in fat and saturated fat will help control the amount of cholesterol in the body. It is important that a diabetic be aware of these things and implement them in the diet. This book offers guidelines for that diet and provides recipes which we hope will help you maintain that diet.

Joseph Turner Crockett, M.D., L.F.A.P.A.
San Diego, California

Chapter 1

DIABETES

Diabetes is a very important disease, and it is getting to be more so every day. Diabetes is not something that happens only to other people. One out of twenty people in the United States has some form of diabetes and one out of four families are in some way affected by it. Diabetes cannot be cured at this time, but if it is caught in time and treated properly, a diabetic can live a long and happy life. Many scientists are hopeful that some method of prevention or cure will be discovered in the next few years.

There are several different types of diabetes:

1. Type I, insulin-dependent (formerly called juvenile-onset) diabetes, is generally found in children and young adults. It usually appears all at once and progresses rapidly. Patients with Type I diabetes need to take insulin because their bodies produce little or no insulin, which they need to maintain utilization of glucose in their body.
2. Type II, non-insulin-dependent (formerly called adult-onset) diabetes, usually occurs in overweight adults forty years or older. It is generally controlled by weight loss, diet and some-

times oral medication. In this type of diabetes, some insulin is produced but it isn't utilized effectively. It can often be prevented or cured if the patient returns to a normal weight and takes regular exercise.

3. Gestational diabetes occurs in some pregnant women and can be controlled by diet. Although most of these women return to normal after their babies are born, it is an indication that they need to watch their weight and get regular exercise, because a great percentage of these women will develop diabetes later in life.
4. Impaired glucose tolerance (formerly called latent diabetes) is diagnosed when a patient's blood sugar levels are between normal and diabetic. This condition can be treated by diet and weight loss to prevent actual diabetes later in life.
5. Secondary diabetes can be caused by drugs or chemicals as well as by pancreatic or endocrine disease.

The warning signs of diabetes are:

Type I	*Type II*
Frequent urination	Excess weight
Abnormal thirst	Drowsiness
Unusual hunger	Blurred vision
Weight loss	Tingling and numbness in hands and feet
Irritability	Skin infections
Weakness or fatigue	Slow healing of cuts, especially on the feet
Nausea and vomiting	Itching, particularly in the vaginal area

When it is discovered that you have diabetes, your doctor will discuss your diet with you or will send you to a registered dietitian who will explain your diet to you. Don't let a doctor send you off with just a sheet of paper with instructions to follow that diet. Each person's diet should be written for their age, weight, physical condition, life style and eating habits, and it can only be written on an individual basis. A diabetic diet is not all that easy to follow and you need specialized instructions. I'm lucky that my doctor, Susan Urbatsch, M.D., from our local clinic at West Union, Iowa, is marvelous with new diabetics and knows that even a registered dietitian needs help coping with other things besides her diet when she becomes diabetic. In the final analysis, a great deal depends upon you and your willingness to learn and cooperate in standardizing your diet . . . and you need to be willing to follow the diet after it is written.

Many doctors don't have the time or the inclination to spend time on your diet, but they can and should recommend a dietitian who can help you. If your doctor doesn't recommend a registered dietitian, ask at the hospital for help, or contact a registered dietitian in private practice. If they aren't available you can call your local nursing home and see if their registered dietitian is willing to help you. Many nursing homes offer this service for good public relations. Make sure that the person who helps you is a registered dietitian or a nutritionist and don't ever, ever let someone who isn't qualified do your diet.

Once you find a registered dietitian, be perfectly frank with her. Tell her what you like to eat and when. If you are a morning person and want a big breakfast but don't care for a snack at night, tell her so. If your budget is tight and you have to watch your pennies, tell her that also. If you like to cook and are willing to make special food for your diet, tell her that, but also tell her if you hate to cook and want as simple a diet as possible. Tell her if you work and carry a lunch with you or if you are dependent upon restaurants for your lunch. (I would recommend that you carry your own lunch to work, if possible.) Help her to help you plan a diet which will fit your life-style and budget as well as your capabilities.

Diabetes can be a very lonesome disease. When you first discover you have diabetes, it can make you feel as though you are all alone in the world. That first period, when you are trying to follow your diet, cope with insulin shots (if necessary), establish an exercise program and lose weight (if necessary), can be overwhelming. I remember how I cried when I discovered I was diabetic and thought that I'd never have any fun or be able to cook anything I liked again. It was hard on me and doubly hard on my husband, whose mother had died of diabetic complications. Life was pretty grim around our house for awhile but you learn to cope with it and discover that there really is life after diabetes.

Now that I have had diabetes for a number of years and have learned how to cope with it, I always tell new diabetics that one of the biggest helps, next to a supportive family, is a group of people who also have diabetes and know how you feel. In fact, you'll probably find that a lot of them are much worse off than you are, and that is a little consolation even if it is getting it the hard way. The best way to find this group of people who can be so supportive is to join your local chapter of the American Diabetes Association. Your doctor or registered dietitian can tell you how to contact the local association. If you don't have a local association, you may need to find one in a neighboring town or start one yourself. If you aren't able to find one, write to

The American Diabetes Association, Inc.
National Service Center
1660 Duke Street
Alexandria, VA 22314.

They will give you the address of your state association who can in turn let you know about the nearest chapter. When you do find a chapter, attend the meetings. Many people refuse to attend meetings because they aren't willing to admit they are diabetic. This is nonsense and only harmful to you. You should not only attend meetings but you should become active in the chapter, if possible, and be there to talk to other diabetics. Offer to help with the annual bike ride (my husband and I have and it is really fun), or make yourself useful in other ways, and you will begin to feel that you aren't all alone and there is a group of people who care and are trying to help each other and you.

After you join the American Diabetes Association, you will receive *Forecast,* a national magazine devoted to promoting the search for a preventive and cure for diabetes and to improving the well-being of people with diabetes and their families. The magazine has some wonderful articles and I find it a real help. You can also subscribe to *DITN (Diabetes in the News),* another publication devoted to serving diabetics and their families around the world. *DITN* may be obtained by writing to:

DITN
1165 N. Clark Street, Suite 311
Chicago, IL 60610

Both magazines have many articles, information and recipes for the diabetic and can be very helpful to you. The state Diabetic Association can be a good source for pamphlets, lists and other helpful information.

Your local library can also be a good source of information, and most hospitals in larger cities have a regular diabetic education program which offers information on preparing diabetic foods and other phases of a diabetic diet. Don't feel bewildered about the whole thing. Get out and get some information and then use it to make your life easier and better.

Chapter 2

FIBER IN THE DIABETIC DIET

Once again our mothers and grandmothers are right. They kept telling us to eat our roughage and now it seems everyone is telling us the same thing. Our grandmothers didn't call it fiber, but that is what they were talking about.

Research is showing us now that fiber, which is the indigestible part of plant foods, can be very helpful in many ways. Of course we all know that a high fiber diet, along with plenty of liquid, will help prevent constipation, but it is only in the last few years we have discovered fiber will do a lot more than prevent constipation. A good amount of fiber, along with plenty of liquid, will, according to the latest research, help control our blood sugar and cholesterol levels as well as help prevent cancer of the colon and diverticulitis.

Sometimes you read about crude fiber and sometimes you read about dietary fiber. Crude fiber is measured by a method using acid and gives the lowest count of fiber content. Dietary fiber is measured by other methods and the count is usually much higher than the count for crude fiber. Most people feel that the count for dietary fiber is much more realistic and includes more of the fiber actually in the food.

There are several different kinds of fiber and they vary according to their source. Grains contain cellulose, hemicellulose and lignin. Fruits and vegetables contain cellulose and pectin, and nuts and seeds contain cellulose and lignin. Meat, poultry, starches, eggs, milk and milk products and refined sugars have little or no fiber. Unfortunately, a lot of fiber is removed when foods are processed in an effort to make them taste better. That is what happened when white flour became common in the last century and eveyone cut the fiber they had been getting for centuries from whole grain flours out of their diets.

Fiber is not a nutrient and therefore provides no calories. It goes through the body basically unchanged, although it does swell and expand with the absorption of liquid. It is this swelling and expansion which adds bulk in the bowels and helps prevent constipation.

There are two theories regarding how fiber helps control blood sugar. One theory is that a diet that is high in fiber is very filling and therefore a diabetic doesn't eat as much food. The other theory is that fiber slows down the absorption of sugar in the bowels and thus helps control the blood sugar levels.

It is important to understand that it is a question of *adequate* fiber, rather than a desire to add as much fiber to the diet as possible. We also need protein and a little fat along with our fruits and vegetables for a well balanced diet. If you aren't used to eating a lot of high fiber foods, it is best to add dietary fiber gradually to your diet. Don't go all out for bran cereal and eat it three times a day. It is much better to increase your intake of fiber gradually and by sensible additions to your diet.

People frequently ask exactly how much dietary fiber they need. Unfortunately, this is difficult to answer. Everyone varies in their need for fiber just as they do for calories and nutrients. So much depends upon age, physical condition and other factors, which makes it difficult to establish any hard-and-fast rules. Most authorities give a ballpark figure with upper and lower limits, but even the authorities disagree, and everyone admits that the information regarding the dietary fiber content of various foods is far from complete at this time. The professionals who have been working on revising *Handbook No. 8,* which is the most authoritative collection of nutritive information, from The United States Department of Agriculture Science and Education Administration, say that it will be some time yet before the information regarding the dietary fiber values of different foods is complete. When it is finally complete and published, it will be much simpler to help people determine how much dietary fiber they need.

However, there is one point on which everyone agrees, and that is that dietary fiber is a very real and important part of our well being and it is important that we consume whatever amount fills our own needs best.

It may sound difficult to increase the fiber content of our diets but in fact, it is very simple. I always advise people that they can increase their dietary fiber intake very easily by making some simple changes in their diet:

1. Change from white bread to whole grain breads.
2. Eat increased amounts of fruits and vegetables.
3. Decrease consumption of highly refined foods such as white flour, sugar (I hope you have already taken care of that) and junk foods.
4. Read labels and use cereals with a higher fiber content.
5. Increase liquid intake to 6 to 8 cups of liquid daily, because liquid is very necessary if fiber is to be used efficiently.

Research indicates that most diabetics respond best to a diet which is higher in complex carbohydrates and lower in fat than was formerly considered advisable. The diabetic food plan used in this book (see Chapter 4) is based on one developed by the Iowa State Dietetic Association and follows those guidelines. Complex carbohydrates are those carbohydrates found in grains, fruits, vegetables and nuts, rather than sugars. These foods also supply dietary fiber along with the carbohydrates, and are helpful in controlling cholesterol as well as blood sugar.

One interesting thought about dietary fiber is that it isn't always where we think it would be. Cabbage is higher in fiber than lettuce and pears contain more fiber than peaches. Any dried peas, beans or lentils are high in fiber and should be used whenever possible. The following lists should be helpful to you in deciding which foods you want to use for a good supply of fiber. Within a few years researchers will be able to give us a more exact list of dietary fiber, but in the meantime, we can be sure of the crude fiber content of the following items even though we aren't positive of their exact dietary fiber content.

Very Good Source of Fiber

Apples with peel
Avocados
Beans of any kind
Berries of any kind
Bran cereals, wheat and oat
Broccoli
Bulgur
Cabbage
Chick peas or garbanzo beans
Cranberries
Figs
Greens of any kind such as mustard, dandelion, kale, turnip
Ground-cherries
Prunes
Pumpkin
Salsify
Soybeans
Winter squash

Good Source of Fiber

Apples, peeled
Applesauce
Apricots
Asparagus
Beets
Bread, whole wheat
Carrots
Cauliflower
Celery
Coconut
Corn and cornmeal
Eggplant
Kumquats
Mangos
Mushrooms
Oatmeal
Pears
Peas
Peppers
Popcorn, popped

Potatoes with skins
Radishes
Raisins
Sauerkraut
Sprouts of soybeans, mung beans, etc.
Sweet potatoes and yams
Tangerines and tangelos
Turnips
Whole grain breads and flours
Wheat germ

Fair Source of Fiber
Cantaloupe and other melons
Cucumbers
Lettuce
Nuts of any kind
Onions
Oranges
Peaches
Potatoes without skins
Summer squash
Tomatoes

I would like to call your attention especially to water-soluble fiber, which seems to be more helpful in controlling blood sugar and cholesterol. Water-soluble fiber is found in oat bran, barley, fruits and legumes (dried peas, beans and lentils). This does not mean we should ignore water-insoluble fiber, which is also helpful in controlling blood sugar, constipation (that certainly makes you feel better) and certain types of cancer, but it does mean we should try to include a good deal of the water-soluble fiber in our diets. We already have a lot of fruit in our diet plans and we should also try to include barley and legumes whenever possible.

Oat bran cereal, which is comparatively new to the market, is particularly good for you. At first it was only available in health food stores, but research has shown it to be so valuable that many people, including me, have pressured their stores until now it is available in most supermarkets. If your store doesn't have it, ask them to get it for you. It can be eaten as a hot cereal or it can be used in other ways. I have included recipes for its use in pie crust, bread, muffins and cookies in this book and I'm sure you will find many other uses for it. If you don't care for it as a hot cereal, you can add a couple of Tablespoons of it to your favorite hot cereal and add some fiber without changing the taste of the cereal. I also find I can use it in many of my favorite recipes which use wheat bran by using half oat bran and half wheat bran equal to the amount of wheat bran listed in the recipe.

A discussion of dried peas, beans and lentils is included in the vegetable chapter (Chapter 8).

Chapter 3

FOOD EXCHANGES

Diabetics have trouble utilizing the carbohydrate in their food because the body either doesn't have enough insulin (Type I) or doesn't utilize insulin correctly (Type II). Because of this, you have to be careful what you eat and count the amount of carbohydrate in it before you eat it. Your doctor or registered dietitian will explain to you how much food (the number of food exchanges) you should eat each day depending upon your type of diabetes, age, weight, height, general health and activity. Almost all Type II diabetics are overweight when they discover they have diabetes and they are generally put on a low calorie diet but most Type I diabetics are more slender and therefore generally get a more liberal diet.

Because the amount of carbohydrate consumed is so important, The American Dietetic Association and the American Diabetes Association, Inc. have established a table classifying various types of foods according to their carbohydrate content along with their protein, fat and caloric values. Each of the classifications is called a food exchange and your doctor or registered dietitian will tell you how many of each exchange you can have during the day.

CONTENT OF FOOD EXCHANGES

Food exchange	Carbohydrate gm.	Protein gm.	Fat gm.	Calories
Starch/bread	15	3	trace	80
Meat: lean		7	3	55
medium-fat		7	5	75
high-fat		7	8	100
Vegetable	5	2		25
Fruit	15			60
Milk: Skim; very low-fat	12	8	1	90
low-fat	12	8	5	120
whole	12	8	8	150
Fat				45

As you can see from the table, one slice of bread contains 15 grams (about 1/2 ounce) of carbohydrate; a serving of fruit, 15 grams of carbohydrate; and a serving of vegetable, 5 grams of carbohydrate. This explains why your doctor or dietitian tells you to eat lots of vegetables and less bread.

It is important to understand that when your dietitian says you can have two bread exchanges at a meal she means that you have two choices from the list of bread exchanges. You could have two slices of bread and use them for a sandwich, or you could have one slice of bread and another choice, such as a baked potato or 1/2 cup of the higher carbohydrate vegetables on the list (e.g., corn or lima beans) . . . or you can skip the bread and have the potato *and* the vegetable. The choice is up to you. That is why they are called exchanges, because you can exchange one food on the list for another one.

This is also true for milk, fruit and vegetable exchanges. If you are allowed two fruit exchanges, you can choose two different servings or double your serving unit using, perhaps, one full cup of orange juice instead of 1/2 cup for breakfast. Most people use two or three ounces of the same kind of meat for a meal although you can always use one or two ounces of meat and one ounce of cheese for a sandwich, or one ounce each of meat, cheese, fish or poultry along with one egg for a big chef's salad.

Research has shown that a diabetic diet which is higher in complex carbohydrates and lower in fat is more successful than the older diabetic diets which included more fat and restricted the use of carbohydrates to a much lower level. Fruits and vegetables should be included in your diet along with whole grain cereals, breads, rice, lentils, dried beans and peas. They are all good sources of complex carbohydrates. A meal pattern based on a high complex-carbohydrate diet is included in Chapter 4. That meal pattern is based on the 1986 food exchange values established by a committee of the American Dietetic and American Diabetes Associations.

The following exchange lists are the basis of a meal planning system designed by a committee of the American Diabetes Association, Inc., and the American Dietetic Association. While designed primarily for people with diabetes and others who must follow special diets, the exchange lists are based on principles of good nutrition and apply to everyone. The lists are copyrighted by the American Diabetes Association, Inc., and the American Dietetic Association, and cannot be reprinted without their permission.

Starch/Bread List Each item in this list contains approximately 15 grams of carbohydrate, 3 grams of protein, a trace of fat and 80 calories. Whole grain products average about 2 grams of fiber per serving. Some foods are higher in fiber. Those foods that contain 3 or more grams of fiber per serving are identified with an asterisk (*).

You can choose your starch exchanges from any of the items on this list. If you want to eat a starch food that is not on this list, the general rule is that 1/2 cup of cereal, grain or pasta is one serving and 1 ounce of bread is one serving. Your dietitian can help you be more exact.

Cereals/Grains/Pasta:

Bran cereals*, concentrated	1/3 cup
Bran cereals*, flaked	1/2 cup
Bulgur, cooked	1/2 cup
Cereals, cooked	1/2 cup
Cereal, puffed	1 1/2 cups
Cereals, ready-to-eat, unsweetened, other	3/4 cup
Cornmeal, dry	2 1/2 Tablespoons
Grapenuts	3 Tablespoons
Grits, cooked	1/2 cup
Pasta, cooked	1/2 cup
Rice, brown and white, cooked	1/3 cup
Wheat, shredded	1/2 cup
Wheat germ*	3 Tablespoons

Dried Beans, Peas, Lentils:

Beans* and Peas*, cooked (kidney, white, split, blackeye)	1/3 cup
Lentils*, cooked	1/3 cup
Beans*, baked	1/4 cup

Starchy Vegetables:

Corn*	1/2 cup
Corn on cob, 6″ long*	1 ear
Green peas*, canned or frozen	1/2 cup
Lima beans*	1/2 cup
Plantain*	1/2 cup
Potato, baked	1 small (3 ounces)
Potatoes, mashed	1/2 cup
Winter squash, acorn, butternut*	3/4 cup
Yams or sweet potatoes, plain	1/3 cup

Bread:

Bagel	1/2 (1 ounce)
Crisp bread sticks, 4″ × 1/2″	2 (2/3 ounce)
Croutons, low-fat	1 cup
English muffin	1/2
Frankfurter or hamburger bun	1/2 (1 ounce)
Pita bread, 6-inch	1/2
Raisin bread, plain	1 slice (1 ounce)
Roll, plain	1 small (1 ounce)
Rye* or pumpernickel* bread	1 slice (1 ounce)
Tortilla, 6-inch	1
White bread, including French and Italian	1 slice (1 ounce)
Whole wheat bread	1 slice (1 ounce)

Crackers and Snacks:

Animal crackers	8
Graham crackers	3 (2 1/2″ square)
Matzoth	3/4 ounce
Melba toast	5 slices
Oyster crackers	24
Popped popcorn	3 cups
Pretzels	3/4 ounce
RyKrisp	4 (2 × 3 1/2 inch)
Saltine-type crackers	6
Whole wheat crackers without added fat (crisp breads such as Finn, Kavli, Wasa)	2 to 4 slices (3/4 ounce)

Starch Foods Prepared with Fat:

(Count as 1 starch/bread serving plus 1 fat serving.)

Biscuits, each 2 1/2 inches across	1
Chow mein noodles	1/2 cup

Corn bread	1 2-inch cube (2 ounces)
Cracker, round butter-type	6
French-fried potatoes, 2- to 3 1/2-inches long	10 (1 1/2 ounces)
Muffin, plain small	1
Pancake, 4″ across	2
Stuffing, bread, prepared	1/4 cup
Taco shell, 6-inch	2
Waffle, 4 1/2″ square	1
Whole wheat crackers with added fat (such as Triscuits)	4 to 6 (1 ounce)

Meat List Each serving of meat or meat substitute on this list contains about 7 grams of protein. The amount of fat and number of calories varies depending upon what kind of meat or substitute you choose. The list is divided into three parts based on the amount of fat and calories: lean meat, medium-fat meat and high-fat meat. One ounce (1 meat exchange) of each of these includes:

	Carbohydrate gm.	*Protein gm.*	*Fat gm.*	*Calories*
Lean	0	7	3	55
Medium-fat	0	7	5	75
High-fat	0	7	8	100

You are encouraged to use more lean and medium-fat meat, poultry and fish in your meal plan. This will help decrease your fat intake, which may help decrease your risk of heart disease. The items from the high-fat group are high in saturated fat, cholesterol, and calories. You should limit your choices from the high-fat group to three (3) times per week. Meat and meat substitutes do not contribute any fiber to your meal plan.

Tips:

1. Bake, roast, broil, grill, or boil these foods rather than frying them with added fat.
2. Use a nonstick pan spray or a nonstick pan to brown or fry these foods.
3. Trim off visible fat before and after cooking.
4. Do not add flour, bread crumbs, coating mixes, or fat to these foods when preparing them.
5. Weigh meat after removing bones and fat, and after cooking. Three ounces of cooked meat is about equal to 4 ounces of raw meat. Some examples of meat portions are:

2 ounces meat (2 meat exchanges)	=	1 small chicken leg or thigh
		1/2 cup cottage cheese or tuna
3 ounces meat (3 meat exchanges)	=	1 medium pork chop
		1 small hamburger
		1/2 of a whole chicken breast
		1 unbreaded fish fillet
		Cooked meat about the size of a deck of cards

6. Restaurants usually serve prime cuts of meat, which are high in fat and calories.

Meats and meat substitutes that have 400 milligrams or more of sodium per exchange are indicated by a dagger (†).

Lean Meat and Substitutes:
(One exchange is equal to any one of the following items)

Beef:	USDA Good or Choice grades of lean beef, such as round, sirloin, and flank steak; tenderloin and chipped beef	1 ounce

Pork:	Lean pork such as fresh ham; canned, cured or boiled ham†, Canadian bacon†, tenderloin	1 ounce
Veal:	All cuts are lean except for veal cutlets (ground or cubed). Examples of lean veal are chops and roasts	1 ounce
Poultry:	Chicken, turkey, Cornish hen (without skin)	1 ounce
Fish:	All fresh and frozen fish	1 ounce
	Crab, lobster, scallops, shrimp, clams (fresh or canned in water)	2 ounces
	Oysters	6 medium
	Tuna† (canned in water) or salmon† (canned in water)	1/4 cup
	Herring (not creamed or smoked)	1 ounce
	Sardines (canned)	2 medium
Game:	Venison, rabbit, squirrel, pheasant, duck, goose (without skin)	1 ounce
Cheese:	Any cottage cheese	1/4 cup
	Grated Parmesan	2 Tablespoons
	Diet cheeses† with less than 55 calories per ounce	1 ounce
Other:	95 percent fat-free luncheon meat†	1 ounce
	Egg whites	3 whites
	Egg substitutes with less than 55 calories per 1/4 cup	1/4 cup

Medium-Fat Meat and Substitutes

(One exchange is equal to any one of the following items.)

Beef:	Most beef products fall into this category. Examples are: all ground beef, roast (rib, chuck, rump), steak (cubed, porterhouse, T-bone) and meatloaf	1 ounce
Pork:	Most pork products fall into this category. Examples are: chops, loin roast, Boston Butt, cutlets	1 ounce

Lamb:	Most lamb products fall into this category. Examples are: chops, leg and roast	1 ounce
Veal:	Cutlet (ground or cubed, unbreaded)	1 ounce
Poultry:	Chicken (with skin), domestic duck or goose (well drained of fat), ground turkey	1 ounce
Fish:	Tuna† (canned in oil and drained) and salmon (canned)	1/4 cup
Cheese:	Skim- or part-skim milk cheese, such as:	
	ricotta	1/4 cup
	mozzarella	1 ounce
	Diet cheeses† with 56–80 calories per ounce	1 ounce
Other:	89 percent fat-free luncheon meats	1 ounce
	Egg (high in cholesterol, limit to 3 per week)	1
	Egg substitutes with 56–80 calories per 1/4 cup	1/4 cup
	Tofu (2 1/2″ × 2 3/4″ × 1″ cube	4 ounces
	Liver, heart, kidneys, sweetbreads (high in cholesterol)	1 ounce

High-Fat Meat and Substitutes

Remember, these items are high in saturated fat, cholesterol, and calories and should be used only three (3) times per week. (One exchange is equal to any one of the following items.)

Beef:	Most USDA Prime cuts of beef, such as ribs or corned beef†	1 ounce
Pork:	Spareribs, ground pork, pork sausage† (patty or link)	1 ounce
Lamb:	Patties (ground lamb)	1 ounce
Fish:	Any fried fish product	1 ounce
Cheese:	All regular cheese† such as American, blue cheddar, Monterey, Swiss	1 ounce

Other:	Luncheon meat† (bologna, salami, pimiento loaf)	1 ounce
	Sausage† (Polish, Italian, knockwurst, [smoked], bratwurst)	1 ounce
	Frankfurter† (turkey or chicken)	1 frank (ten to the pound)
	Peanut butter (contains unsaturated fat)	1 Tablespoon

Count as 1 high-fat meat plus 1 fat exchange:

Frankfurter† (beef, pork or combination)	1 frank (ten to the pound)

Vegetable List Each vegetable serving on this list contains about 5 grams of carbohydrate, 2 grams of protein and 25 calories. Vegetables contain 2–3 grams of dietary fiber. Vegetables which contain 400 milligrams or more of sodium per serving are identified by a dagger (†).

Vegetables are a good source of vitamins and minerals. Fresh and frozen vegetables have more vitamins and less added salt. Rinsing canned vegetables will remove much of the salt.

Unless otherwise noted, the serving size for vegetables (one vegetable exchange) is 1/2 cup cooked vegetables or vegetable juice, or 1 cup of raw vegetables.

1/2 medium artichoke
Asparagus
Beans (green, wax or Italian)
Bean sprouts
Beets
Broccoli
Brussels sprouts
Cabbage, cooked
Carrots
Cauliflower
Eggplant
Greens (collard, mustard, turnip)
Kohlrabi
Leeks
Mushrooms, cooked
Okra
Onions
Pea pods
Peppers, green
Rutabega

Sauerkraut†
Spinach, cooked
Summer squash, crookneck
Tomato, one large
Tomato vegetable juice†
Turnips
Water chestnuts
Zucchini, cooked

Free Vegetables:
You can eat as much as you like of the items for which no serving size is specified. You may eat two or three servings per day of those items that have a specified serving size. Be sure to spread these servings out through the day.

Cabbage, raw, 1 cup
Celery, raw, 1 cup
Chinese cabbage*, raw, 1 cup
Cucumber
Green onions
Hot peppers
Mushrooms
Radishes
Salad greens (endive, escarole, lettuce, romaine, spinach)
Zucchini

Starchy vegetables such as corn, peas and potatoes are found on the Starch/Bread List.

Fruit List Each item on this list contains about 15 grams of carbohydrate and 60 calories. Fresh, frozen and dry fruits have about 2 grams of fiber per serving. Fruits that have 3 or more grams of fiber per serving are identified with an asterisk (*).

The carbohydrate and calorie content for a fruit serving are based on the usual serving of the most commonly eaten fruits. Use fresh fruits or fruits frozen without added sugar. Whole fruit is more filling than fruit juice and may be a better choice for those who are trying to lose weight. Unless otherwise noted, the serving size for one fruit serving is 1/2 cup of fresh fruit or fruit juice, or 1/4 cup dried fruit.

Fresh, frozen and unsweetened canned fruit:

Apple, raw, 2 inches across	1 apple
Applesauce, unsweetened	1/2 cup
Apricots, raw, medium	4 apricots
Apricots, canned	1/2 cup or 4 halves
Banana, 9 inches long	1/2
Blackberries*, raw	3/4 cup
Blueberries*, raw	3/4 cup
Cantaloupe, 5 inches across	1/3
Cantaloupe cubes, raw	1 cup
Cherries, raw, large	12 cherries
Cherries, canned	1/2 cup
Figs, raw, 2 inches across	2 figs
Fruit cocktail, canned	1/2 cup
Grapefruit, medium	1/2 grapefruit
Grapefruit segments	3/4 cup
Grapes, small	15 grapes
Honeydew melon, medium	1/8 melon
Honeydew melon cubes	1 cup
Kiwi, large	1 kiwi
Mandarin oranges	3/4 cup
Mango, small	1/2 mango
Nectarine*, 1 1/2 inches across	1 nectarine
Orange, 2 1/2 inches across	1 orange
Papaya	1 cup
Peach, 2 3/j4 inches across	1 peach or 3/4 cup
Peaches, canned	1/2 cup or 2 halves
Pear	1/2 large or 1 small
Pears, canned	1/2 cup or 2 halves
Native persimmon, medium	2 persimmons
Pineapple, raw	3/4 cup
Pineapple, canned	1/3 cup
Plum, raw, 2 inches across	2 plums
Pomegranate*	1/2 pomegranate
Raspberries*, raw	1 cup
Strawberries*, raw, whole	1 1/4 cups
Tangerine, 2 1/2 inches across	2 tangerines
Watermelon cubes	1 1/4 cups

Dried fruit:

Apples*	4 rings
Apricots*	7 halves
Dates, medium	2 1/2 dates
Figs*	1 1/2
Prunes*, medium	3
Raisins	2 Tablespoons

Fruit juice:

Apple juice/cider	1/2 cup
Cranberry juice cocktail	1/3 cup
Grape juice	1/3 cup
Grapefruit juice	1/2 cup
Orange juice	1/2 cup
Pineapple juice	1/2 cup
Prune juice	1/3 cup

Free Fruits:
You may have two or three servings per day of these items. Be sure to spread the servings out through the day.

Cranberries, unsweetened	1/2 cup
Rhubarb, unsweetened	1/2 cup

Milk List Each serving of milk or milk products on this list contains about 12 grams of carbohydrate and 8 grams of protein. The amount of fat in milk is measured in percent (%) of butterfat. The calories vary depending on what kind of milk you choose. The list is divided into three parts based on the amount of fat and calories: skim/very lowfat milk, lowfat milk, and whole milk. One serving (1 milk exchange) of each of these includes:

	Carbohydrate gm.	*Protein gm.*	*Fat gm.*	*Calories*
Skim/very lowfat	12	8	trace	90
Lowfat	12	8	5	120
Whole	12	8	8	150

Milk is the body's main source of calcium, the mineral needed for growth and repair of bones. Yogurt is also a good source of calcium. Yogurt and many dry or powdered milk products have different amounts of fat. If you have questions about a particular item, read the label to find out the fat and calorie content.

Milk is good to drink, but it can also be added to cereal and other foods. Many tasty dishes such as sugar-free pudding are made with milk (see combination foods list, page 38). Add life to plain yogurt by adding one of your fruit servings to it.

Skim and very lowfat milk:

Skim milk	1 cup
1/2% milk	1 cup
1% milk	1 cup
Lowfat buttermilk	1 cup
Evaporated skim milk	1/2 cup
Dry nonfat milk	1/3 cup
Plain nonfat yogurt	8 ounces

Lowfat Milk:

2% milk	1 cup
Plain lowfat yogurt with added nonfat milk solids	8 ounces

Whole milk:

Whole milk	1 cup
Evaporated whole milk	1/2 cup
Whole plain yogurt	8 ounces

Fat List Each serving on the fat list contains about 5 grams fat and 45 calories.

The foods on the fat list contain mostly fat, although some items may also contain a small amount of protein. All fats are high in calories and should be carefully measured. Everyone should modify fat intake by eating unsaturated fats instead of saturated fats. The sodium content of these foods varies widely. Check the label for sodium information.

Some foods have a sodium content of over 400 milligrams if more than one or two servings are used. These foods are indicated by a double dagger(‡).

Unsaturated fats:

Avocado	1/8 medium
Margarine	1 teaspoon
Margarine‡, diet	1 Tablespoon
Mayonnaise‡, reduced-calorie	1 Tablespoon
Mayonnaise-type salad dressing	2 teaspoons
Mayonnaise-type salad dressing, reduced-calorie	1 Tablespoon
Nuts and seeds	
Dry roasted almonds	6 whole
Dry roasted cashews	1 Tablespoon
Peanuts	20 small or 10 large
Pecans	2 whole
Pine nut seeds	1 Tablespoon
Pumpkin seeds	2 teaspoons
Sunflower seeds (without shells)	1 Tablespoon
Walnuts	2 whole
Other nuts	1 Tablespoon
Oil—corn, cottonseed, olive, safflower, soybean or sunflower	1 teaspoon
Olives‡	10 small or 5 large
Salad dressing	1 Tablespoon
Salad dressing, low-calorie	Up to 2 Tablespoons is a free food
Salad dressing, reduced-calorie	2 Tablespoons

Saturated Fats:

Butter	1 teaspoon
Bacon‡	1 slice
Chitterlings	1/2 ounce

Shredded coconut	2 Tablespoons
Liquid coffee whitener	2 Tablespoons
Dry coffee whitener	4 teaspoons
Light, coffee or table cream	2 Tablespoons
Sour cream	2 Tablespoons
Heavy or whipping cream	1 Tablespoon
Cream cheese	1 Tablespoon
Salt pork‡	1/4 ounce

Free Foods A free food is any food or drink that contains less than 20 calories per serving. You can eat as much as you want of items that have no serving size specified. You may eat two or three servings per day of items that have a specified serving size. Be sure to spread them out through the day.

Drinks:

Bouillon† or fat-free broth
Low-sodium bouillon
Sugar-free carbonated drinks
Club soda or mineral water
Unsweetened cocoa powder (1 Tablespoon)
Coffee or tea
Sugar-free drink mixes
Sugar-free tonic water
Nonstick pan spray

Free fruits and vegetables are listed under the appropriate headings.

Sweet Substitutes:

Sugar-free hard candy
Sugar-free gelatin
Sugar-free gum
Sugar-free jams and jellies (2 teaspoons)
Sugar-free pancake syrup (1/4 cup)
Sugar substitutes such as saccharin and aspartame
Low-calorie whipped topping

Condiments:

Catsup (1 Tablespoon)
Dill pickles, unsweetened
Horseradish
Mustard
Salad dressing, low-calorie (up to 2 Tablespoons is free)
Taco sauce (1 Tablespoon)
Vinegar

Seasonings:
Seasonings can be very helpful in making food taste better. Be careful of how much sodium is used. Read the label and choose those seasonings which do not contain sodium or salt.

Basil, fresh
Celery seeds
Chili powder
Chives
Cinnamon
Curry
Dill
Flavoring extracts such as almond, butter, lemon, peppermint, vanilla, walnut
Garlic
Garlic powder
Herbs
Hot pepper sauce
Lemon or lemon juice
Lemon pepper
Lime or lime juice
Mint
Onion powder
Oregano
Paprika
Pepper
Pimiento
Spices
Soy sauce†
Soy sauce, low-sodium or "Lite"
Wine used for cooking (1/4 cup)
Worcestershire sauce

Combination Foods Much of the food we eat is mixed together in various combinations. These combination foods fit into more than one exchange list. It can be quite hard to tell what is in a certain casserole or baked food item. This is a list of average values for some typical combination foods. This list will help you fit these foods into your meal plan. Ask your dietitian for information about other foods you'd like to eat.

The American Diabetes Association/American Dietetic Association Family Cookbooks and *The American Diabetes Association Holiday Cookbook* have many recipes and further information about many foods, including combination foods. Check your library or local bookstore for these and other diabetic cookbooks.

Food	*Exchanges*
8-ounce cup of homemade casserole	2 starch, 2 medium-fat meat, 1 fat
1/4 of 15-ounce or 10-inch thin-crust cheese pizza†	2 starch, 2 medium-fat meat, 1 fat
8-ounce cup of commercial chili with beans*†	2 starch, 2 medium-fat meat, 2 fat
2 cups (16 ounces) chow mein without rice or noodles*‡	1 starch, 2 vegetable, 2 lean meat
8-ounce cup of macaroni and cheese†	2 starch, 1 medium-fat meat, 2 fat
8-ounce cup canned spaghetti and meat balls†	2 starch, 1 medium-fat meat, 1 fat
1/2 cup sugar-free pudding made with skim milk	1 starch
1 cup cooked dried beans*, peas* or lentils*	2 starch, 1 lean meat
Soup	
8-ounce cup beans*†	1 starch, 1 vegetable, 1 lean meat
10 3/4-ounce can all chunky varieties	1 starch, 1 vegetable, 1 medium-fat meat
8-ounce cup cream soup made with water‡	1 starch, 1 fat
8-ounce cup vegetable‡ or broth‡	1 starch

Foods for Occasional Use Moderate amounts of some foods can be used in your meal plan in spite of their sugar or fat content, as long as you can maintain blood-glucose control. The following list includes average exchange values for some of these foods. Because they are concentrated sources of carbohydrate, you will notice that the portion sizes are very small. Check with your dietitian for advice on how often and when you can eat them.

Food	*Exchanges*
1/12 angel food cake	2 starch
3″ square or 1/12 cake without icing	2 starch, 2 fat
2 small cookies, 1 3/4 inches across	1 starch, 1 fat
1/3 cup frozen fruit yogurt	1 starch
3 gingersnaps	1 starch
1/4 cup granola	1 starch, 1 fat
1 small granola bar	1 starch, 1 fat
1/2 cup ice cream, any flavor	1 starch, 2 fat
1/2 cup ice milk, any flavor	1 starch, 1 fat
1/4 cup sherbet, any flavor	1 starch
1 ounce snack chips‡, all varieties	1 starch, 2 fat
6 small vanilla wafers	1 starch, 1 fat

Chapter 4

PLANNING MENUS

I'm sure your doctor or registered dietitian has given you a list of food exchanges which are the basis for your menu planning. That list is planned according to your needs and you should eat everything on the list, but try not to add anything to the list except "free foods" such as free vegetables or salads, diet beverages and coffee or tea.

This chapter includes a food plan based on a high–complex carbohydrate diet. The food plan is based on one included in *The New Simplified Diet Manual* written by the Iowa Dietetic Association with modifications for the new food exchange values. I have been using it for myself and for patients and find it very satisfying. It includes a good supply of fruits and vegetables for fiber and is based on the idea that you will use high fiber breads and cereals whenever possible.

You don't need to worry about getting a balanced diet if your calorie allowance is 1200 calories or more per day. If your allowance is below that, your doctor will probably advise a simple vitamin and mineral supplement. Diets at 1200 calories or more have the basic nutritional needs built into them including:

Two or more servings of meat, poultry or fish per day;
Three or more servings of fruits and vegetables per day;
Three or more servings of whole grain cereals per day; and
Two or more 8-ounce glasses of milk per day.

Sometimes it helps to have a sheet on which you can write the number of exchanges in your meal plan when you are first starting to follow your diabetic meal plan. After you have been planning your diet for awhile, you can do it without a sheet of paper. You can buy some books with charts in them, some drug manufacturers pass out complimentary copies of them, and you can always make your own. I find the following chart helpful for my own use and have given it to patients who reported that it helped them also. Please feel free to have it copied if you'd like. After you have it copied, write the number of exchanges you are allowed for each meal, and then at the end of the meal, write how you have used those exchanges. If your blood sugar is acting up, it is easier to be able to go back and decide exactly why it happened, or at least it will give a good indication of the possible trouble.

Date **How I used my exchanges today**

BREAKFAST:

Starch (bread)

Fruit

Skim milk

Fat

LUNCH OR SUPPER:

Starch/bread

Lean meat

Vegetables

Fruit

Skim milk

Fat

DINNER:

Starch (bread)

Lean meat

Vegetables

Fruit

Skim milk

Fat

SNACK:

Starch (bread)

Fruit

Skim milk

NOTES:

Following is a basic meal pattern for diabetic diets based on a high–complex carbohydrate diet. I have included the percentages of carbohydrate, protein and fat for your information since this diet is based on a higher carbohydrate level than was formerly used.

MEAL PATTERNS FOR DIABETIC DIETS

Calorie Level	*1000*	*1200*	*1500*	*1800*	*2000*
Exchanges					
Starch/bread	3	5	6	8	9
Lean meat	4	5	5	6	6
Vegetables	2	2	2	2	2
Fruits	3	4	5	6	6
Skim milk	2	2	3	3	3
Fat	3	2	3	3	6
Total Calories	*1005*	*1235*	*1510*	*1785*	*2000*
Percentages					
Cho (Carbohydrate)	50	54	56	57	54
Pro (Protein)	23	23	21	21	19
Fat	27	23	23	22	27

When you break this meal pattern down into individual meals, you will generally use the following, although your doctor or registered dietitian might want to change the arrangement somewhat to conform to your own eating patterns.

SAMPLE MENU PATTERNS

Calorie Level	*1000*	*1200*	*1500*	*1800*	*2000*
Breakfast					
Starch (bread)	1	2	2	2	3
Lean meat	0	0	0	0	0
Vegetables	0	0	0	0	0
Fruits	1	1	1	2	2
Skim milk	1/2	1/2	1	1	1
Fat	1	1	1	1	2
Lunch					
Starch (bread)	1	1 1/2	2	2	2
Lean meat	2	2	2	3	3
Vegetables	1	1	1	1	1
Fruits	1	1	1	2	2
Skim milk	1/2	1/2	1	1	1
Fat	1	1/2	1	1	2
Dinner					
Starch (bread)	1	1	1	3	3
Lean meat	2	3	3	3	3
Vegetables	1	1	1	1	1
Fruits	1	1	2	1	1
Skim milk	1/2	1/2	1/2	1/2	1/2
Fat	1	1/2	1	1	2
Snacks					
Starch (bread)	0	1/2	1	1	1
Fruit	0	1	1	1	1
Skim milk	1/2	1/2	1/2	1/2	1/2
Fat	0	0	0	0	0

Chapter 5

INGREDIENTS

Many people think that because a food is labelled "dietetic" or "diabetic" it will fit easily into their diabetic diets or, worse yet, that it is free. This is a misconception that can lead to some pretty high blood sugar counts. The first thing to do when you see foods labeled that way is to read the labels to see exactly what they mean by the word dietetic or diabetic, the size serving they use for their nutritive calculations and how many grams of carbohydrate, protein and fat are in each serving. Remember how many grams of carbohydrate, protein and fat are in the different exchanges and then compare them with the amounts on the label and you will see how many exchanges the food will cost you. If you have difficulty remembering the content of the different exchanges you can carry a little card with you on which the different values are written (see Chapter 3).

Low-calorie foods are a large part of the market these days and the leading packers and manufacturers are beginning to offer foods that are good for diabetics. These foods are often found in the main aisles of the stores and not in a specially marked section. Fruits are available packed in water without sugar or in fruit juice without sugar. The ones packed in fruit juice can be very tasty. Check the label for their carbohydrate value since they are generally higher in carbohydrates than the fruit packed in water without sugar. I generally buy fruit canned in water without sugar. It has a good flavor which is even better if you open it one day, sweeten the juice with Equal and then return it to the refrigerator to marinate overnight before it is eaten.

Fresh fruits or fruits frozen without sugar are also a big plus for your diabetic diet and add fiber, vitamins and minerals as well as taste-appeal to your diet.

There are even some mixes available for diabetic foods. The ones for salad dressings are excellent and can also be used for seasoning other foods. I don't bother with the cake mixes. It is too easy to make your own cake or cookie mix (see Chapter 12) to bother buying a commercial mix.

Many diabetics are also on a low-sodium diet, which used to be really rough. There was almost no help in the stores—but all that has changed now. There is suddenly a wealth of food available for anyone on a low-sodium diet. There are low-sodium soups and canned vegetables and salt-free margarines available as well as salt substitutes. I didn't mention using salt substitutes in recipes because it is not a good idea to use them unless your doctor has given you permission to do so. If your doctor agrees that you can use them, try several different kinds and then choose the one you like best and use it to give added zest to your food. If you don't find a salt substitute you like, you can always substitute herbs and spices as well as lemon juice for additional flavor.

I have included the use of liquid egg substitute in the low-cholesterol variation of many of the recipes. Liquid egg substitute is an excellent product and can be used for many things. My husband is on a low-cholesterol diet and we use a lot of the liquid egg substitute. He even makes luscious omelets out of it and I really like it for Fritatta (see p. 98).

Following is a more detailed discussion of some of the foods used in recipes in this book.

Sugar

Yes, diabetics can use some sugar as long as it is counted in the nutritive analysis. This doesn't mean you can use sugar on your cereal or in your lemonade but it does mean that a small amount of sugar can be used in food preparation. The use of even a small amount of sugar has made a big difference in food preparation particularly of cakes, cookies and other baked goods, because even a little sugar helps the flavor and texture of baked products so much that it is a whole new world of food preparation for diabetics. Be very careful, when measuring sugar for these recipes, to measure it *exactly,* because the recipes have been tested with the amounts given. You could probably give the recipe a little better texture if you increased the sugar, but remember if you do that you are changing the food exchange values and they will no longer be accurate. I make it a policy never to buy any foods which list sugar as an ingredient unless the nutritive values are listed on the container, because you can't be sure how much has been used unless the nutritive analysis is included.

Sometimes the most practical thing is to use a little bit of sugar for texture and then use sugar substitute for the taste of sweetness that we all like.

Sugar Substitutes

Saccharin has been around a long time and has its important uses in baking but I think that many people prefer the taste of Equal (Nutrasweet or aspartame). Equal is marvelous for gelatins and puddings which don't have to be cooked, and I'm sure we all enjoy the taste of a good diet drink occasionally. However, Equal can't be used for baking or any exposure to sustained heat.

I'm not too fond of the taste of sugar substitutes except for Equal so I tend to use a minimum of them. However, if you like more sweetness, feel free to add more of the sugar substitutes. You won't change the food exchanges of the product.

I specified the type of sugar substitutes in recipes only when I felt it was really important to use a particular one, so please use the one specified if at all possible.

Because you will be using a variety of sugar substitutes and because I like to know how much of a particular kind of sugar substitute is equal to a certain amount of sugar, I have included the following table of sugar substitute and sugar equivalents.

Sugar Substitutes and Equivalents

1 teaspoon sugar
- 1 teaspoon Sprinkle Sweet
- 1 teaspoon Sugar Twin
- 1 Equal tablet
- 1/2 packet Equal
- 2 shakes of the Adolph's jar
- 1/10 teaspoon Sweet 'n Low
- 1/8 teaspoon Weight Watchers

1 Tablespoon sugar
- 1 Tablespoon Sprinkle Sweet
- 1 Tablespoon Sugar Twin
- 1 1/2 packets Equal
- 1/4 teaspoon Adolph's
- 1/3 teaspoon Sweet 'n Low
- 3/8 teaspoon Weight Watchers

1/4 cup sugar
- 1/4 cup Sprinkle Sweet
- 1/4 cup Sugar Twin
- 6 packets Equal
- 1 teaspoon Adolph's
- 1 1/2 teaspoons Sweet 'n Low
- 1 1/2 teaspoons Weight Watchers

1/2 cup sugar
- 1/2 cup Sprinkle Sweet
- 1/2 cup Sugar Twin
- 12 packets Equal
- 2 teaspoons Adolph's
- 1 Tablespoon Sweet 'n Low
- 1 Tablespoon Weight Watchers

3/4 cup sugar
- 3/4 cup Sprinkle Sweet
- 3/4 cup Sugar Twin
- 18 packets Equal
- 1 Tablespoon Adolph's
- 1 1/2 Tablespoons Sweet 'n Low
- 1 1/2 Tablespoons Weight Watchers

1 cup sugar
- 1 cup Sprinkle Sweet
- 1 cup Sugar Twin
- 24 packets Equal
- 4 teaspoons Adolph's
- 2 Tablespoons Sweet 'n Low
- 2 Tablespoons Weight Watchers

Instant Dry Milk

I have been using instant dry milk and persuading others to use it for years because of its convenience and economy. It is even more important that we use it now, because it is almost completely fat-free, and while the new complex carbohydrate diet gives us more carbohydrate in our diabetic diet, it also keeps fat exchanges to a minimum.

There are several methods of using instant dry milk and we use most of them in the recipes in this book. I don't believe in reconstituting instant dry milk except for drinking or using on cereal. Other than that, you can generally incorporate the dry milk into the other ingredients very easily. However, if you want to drink the reconstituted milk, you should mix it several hours before it is used so it can be thoroughly chilled. My sister likes to have about 1/2 teaspoon vanilla per quart in her reconstituted milk, which doesn't add any calories or other exchanges. If you want to reconstitute the milk for drinking, follow the directions on the package for skim milk, don't add any butter or other fat to the milk, chill it well and enjoy it with your meals or for a snack.

I have also been using dry buttermilk, which is available at many stores. If your store doesn't carry it, ask them to order it for you. It is much more convenient to have a can of dry buttermilk on hand to use when you need it than it is to have to keep buying fresh buttermilk, and less expensive also. It, too, can be reconstituted but I prefer to use it in with the flour or other ingredients instead of reconstituting it before it is used.

Bran Cereals

Several different kinds of bran cereals are listed in recipes. Feel free to use whichever you prefer, but don't substitute the bran you buy in a health food store, because you won't get the same results. Nutritive values used are an average of the nutritive values of all four of the bran cereals. Bran is a very good source of fiber, and I highly recommend that you use it and the recipes including it often.

I have used oat bran cereal in several recipes. Oat bran cereal cannot be substituted for the bran cereals, but it can be used as a hot cereal or in recipes which specify oat bran. Research indicates that oat bran cereal is as good as, or better than, the wheat bran cereal that we have been using.

Yeast

Quick-rise yeast is used in several recipes. It is a form of active dry yeast which will help the bread to rise more rapidly than it will with the standard quick-rise yeast. Both active dry and quick-rise yeast need to be dissolved in water or other liquid at 110 to 115 degrees and both forms of yeast will die when exposed to heat above 140 degrees.

Vegetable Oil

Vegetable oil is used in many recipes because it helps to lower a cholesterol count and because it is handy to use. Corn and soybean oil are best for everyday use and may be used in any of these recipes.

Margarine

Margarine is used instead of butter because many diabetics have a high cholesterol count which can be lowered by substituting margarine and vegetable oil for butter and lard or other animal fats. Read the label when you are buying margarine and choose only margarines made with vegetable oils such as corn or soybean oil. Do not buy margarines that include lard, palm or coconut oil.

Salt-free margarine is available at most stores and should be used on a low-sodium diet. If your store doesn't have salt-free margarine, they can get it for you easily. You can, if necessary, buy several pounds and freeze it until you need it.

Bouillon

Nutritive values for recipes using bouillon are based on the use of the commercial bouillon cubes which have a high percentage of salt. If you are on a low-sodium diet, buy low-sodium bouillon cubes or powder and you will lower the sodium count on a recipe very quickly. Stock or bouillon which you make without added salt is the best choice, but if you don't have time to do that, the low-sodium commercial bases are good and will help to keep your sodium intake low. Low-sodium bouillon base in both chicken and beef flavor should be available at your store. If you can't get it at the store, ask the manager to get it for you or buy it at a health food store.

Chapter 6

SOUPS

Soup can give you a lot of satisfaction for very few exchanges and can provide fiber and nutrients without adding sugar, fat, cholesterol or much sodium. It always reminds me of home and love and warmth and all those nice things. My mother said she couldn't remember making that much soup but both my sister and I remember it that way, so I guess we were more impressed with her soups than she was.

Most soups are a good source of nutrients, especially vegetable soups. However, you need to choose your soup as wisely as you do all of your food. Fortunately, most commercial soups now have the nutritive information on the label so you know how many exchanges they will cost you. (Isn't that phrase—"cost" you—misleading! I once told a friend of mine that I couldn't afford something and she told me that I'd better go back to work if I couldn't afford that . . . She didn't realize I meant I couldn't afford to spend the exchanges that food item would "cost" me.) I like to use water to thin commercial soups, but if you like to use milk, you will need to count that milk also. If you are counting your sodium intake, I'm sure you are happy to know that there are many low-sodium soups on the market now and they are very good.

I divide soups into three categories when I'm planning meals.

1. Soups which are free, such as clear broth with very little rice or pasta or a few julienned vegetables.
2. Soups with vegetables and meat, fish or chicken, which you might serve with a sandwich for lunch along with a salad and your fruit exchange. These are my favorite soups and I've included several in this chapter.
3. Soups which are luxury items for diabetics, such as those containing quite a bit of beans, potatoes, corn, pasta or other high-carbohydrate foods, with perhaps cream or egg yolks for thickening. If you use these soups, you are generally restricted to salads and fruit with maybe a couple of crackers and a free gelatin, but some of them are so good, they are worth it.

If you want to use your own recipe for a vegetable soup, the broth is free but you must count the vegetables and/or starchy foods you add to the broth as well as any fish, meat or chicken added later. For instance, if you wanted to make a vegetable soup using the following ingredients:

5 cups beef or chicken broth	Free
1/2 cup chopped cooked onions	1 vegetable exchange
1/2 cup chopped cooked carrots	1 vegetable exchange
1/2 cup chopped cooked green beans	1 vegetable exchange
1/2 cup diced cooked white potatoes	1 bread or 3 vegetable exchanges
Total	6 vegetable exchanges

This recipe will yield about 6 cups of soup, so one cup of soup will cost you 1 vegetable exchange. If you want more vegetables in your soup but don't want to increase the cost in exchanges, you can substitute 1 1/2 cups of cooked vegetables such as cabbage, broccoli, or tomatoes or more of the original vegetable list for the 1/2 cup diced potatoes without changing the exchange value of the soup.

If you want meat or chicken in your soup, you can add as much as you like, considering that you will get 6 cups of soup. For instance, if you want to add 1 ounce meat or chicken per serving to the soup, you would add 1 cup (6 ounces) cubed, cooked meat or chicken with fat and gristle removed to the soup after the vegetables are cooked. I like to add 2 ounces (1/3 cup) of the cooked diced meat or chicken to my soup bowl, add 1 cup of the vegetable soup and then add the rest of the meat to the soup for the rest of the family. If I freeze the soup for my own use later, I add the right amount of soup and meat or chicken to each container and then label it "1 vegetable and 1 meat exchange" so I'll know how to count it when I use it at some later date.

When you are preparing just 1 serving of soup for yourself, you can use as much of the free broth as you like and then add 1/2 cup mixed cooked and/or canned vegetables and as much meat as you like for a soup with 1 vegetable exchange plus the meat exchanges. If you want a soup with noodles or rice, you can use the same method, counting 1 bread exchange for each 1/2 cup cooked pasta, noodles or rice.

If you are trying to cut down on your salt (sodium) intake, it is a good idea to prepare your own salt-free broth at home. Both beef and chicken broth depend upon good quality ingredients. I like to use beef or veal for beef broth, and some people like lamb broth. I don't really care for broth made with pork. You can get beef or veal bones from your butcher. I also like to put bones, meat scraps, meat trimmings, etc. in the freezer until I have enough of them to make a good broth. When I have enough to fill my stew pot, I defrost the bones and meat, place them in an open roaster and roast them, uncovered, at 350°F until they are well browned. The browning develops the flavor of the meat and bones and will yield a richer tasting broth. After the bones and meat are browned, put them in a Dutch oven or large stew pot, cover them with cold water and bring to a simmer. Simmer for a few minutes, skim off the scum on top and then add a couple of carrots, a stalk of celery and a chopped onion and simmer, covered, for four to six hours. The broth may look finished to you before four hours but it will be much better if you let it simmer for at least the minimum of four hours. At the end of four to six hours, drain off the broth and refrigerate until the fat has risen to the top and hardened so that it can be removed and discarded. The broth is then ready to be used or frozen, as you desire. The bones should be discarded along with the cooked vegetables and the meat cooled until you can trim off any fat or gristle after which it can be used, or frozen for later use.

Chicken broth is prepared essentially the same way except that the chicken or turkey carcass, back, neck, wings and bones are covered with cold water, simmered for five minutes and then drained. Fresh cold water is added to the chicken, a couple of carrots, a stalk of celery and some onions are added, the pan is covered tightly and the broth is allowed to simmer for two to two and one half hours.

The nicest part of using these homemade broths is that they are very low in sodium. The sodium content of soups in this chapter are calculated using commercial bouillon cubes because that is what most people use. I figure 1 cube per cup of broth with 1,152 mg. of sodium per beef bouillon cube and 1,487 mg. sodium per chicken bouillon cube, so you see you can really cut the sodium in soups by using homemade broths. Many grocery stores are now beginning to stock low-sodium bouillon cubes, which we used to have to buy in health food stores. If your grocery store doesn't carry the low-sodium cubes you can ask the owner or manager to get them for you. Mr. Bostrom, who owns our local Super-Valu store, is very cooperative when I ask him to get something for me. If it sells he keeps it on the shelf and if it doesn't sell he stops carrying it, which I think is fair.

Soup looks more attractive when you add a garnish before you serve it. There are several garnishes which don't take any food exchanges but do make the soup look better, such as a little chopped green onions or chives, a few croutons, a slice of lemon, chopped parsley or even a little popcorn and other goodies which can be used without counting them.

Chuck has taught me to like the Italian way of adding cheese to soup. An ounce of grated cheddar, colby, mozzarella or other cheese that melts well adds a lot to a bowl of soup. The cheese must be added while the soup is hot so it will melt, or you can put it in the microwave oven for a few seconds if necessary.

I used a smaller number of servings for soups that are easy to prepare, and a larger number of servings for the more complicated soups such as minestrone, which can be frozen and used at a later date without going through all of those complicated steps again.

Meat and vegetables should be cut into fairly uniform pieces so they will cook evenly. 1/2- to 1/4-inch cubes are good, but this is a personal decision and you may prefer them larger or julienned. It is a bit of work to cut them all evenly but it yields the best results and is worth the time and trouble.

There are some very good soup mixes on the market. I like to use Lipton's onion soup mix for seasoning as well as for soup. When you prepare the soup according to the directions on the package, 1/4 of the soup will cost you 1/2 bread exchange. If you find a soup mix you like which doesn't provide a nutritional analysis, I would compare it to a known soup and its value. For instance, if you use a soup mix for vegetable soup, you know the broth is free and you can decide about the vegetables. If you have 1/2 cup of high carbohydrate vegetables such as corn, dry beans or potatoes, you know it will be 1 bread exchange, and if it has 1/2 cup of the regular vegetables such as carrots, onions, celery, broccoli or cabbage, it will be 1 vegetable exchange. If you have a soup mix with no analysis and you know it is high carbohydrate, you can compare it with a known soup of the same ingredients, such as a regular split pea soup, which will vary from 1 to 1 1/2 bread exchanges for about 1 cup of soup.

Bean Soup

2 Tablespoons margarine
1/2 cup shredded carrots
1/2 cup onions, chopped fine
4 cups fat-free chicken broth
1 3/4 cups (15-ounce can) canned lima or butter beans
1 cup diced fresh potatoes
1 2/3 cups (10 ounces) diced cooked ham with fat and skin removed
Sprinkle of pepper (optional)

Melt margarine in a 3-quart saucepan over medium heat. Add carrots and onions and cook and stir over medium heat until the vegetables are soft but not browned. Add broth, beans and potatoes to the vegetables, cover and simmer for 20 minutes or until the potatoes are tender. Mash some of the beans and potatoes against the side of the pan with the back of a spoon. Add ham and pepper to the soup, cover and continue to simmer for another 5 minutes. Serve hot, using 1 cup soup per serving.

Nutritive values per serving: *cal 207, cho 16 gm, pro 17 gm, fat 8 gm, Na 1,298 mg. This recipe is a good source of fiber.*

Food exchanges per serving: *1 bread and 2 lean meat*

Low-sodium diets: *Use salt-free margarine, low-sodium broth and beans cooked without salt.*

Low-cholesterol diets: *May be used as written.*

Yield: *1 1/2 quarts, 6 servings*

Beef Barley Soup

3 1/2 cups rich, flavorful beef broth
1/2 cup chopped onions
1/2 cup chopped celery
2 Tablespoons quick-cooking barley
1 teaspoon Worcestershire sauce
1/4 teaspoon garlic powder
salt and pepper to taste
1 cup (6 ounces) cooked, diced lean beef with fat and gristle removed

Combine broth, onions and celery in a 2-quart saucepan, cover and simmer 10 minutes. Add barley to soup and simmer another 10 minutes. Add Worcestershire sauce, garlic powder, salt and pepper to taste. (The amount of salt needed will depend upon the saltiness of the broth.) Cover and simmer another 5 minutes. Serve hot, using 1 cup soup per serving.

Nutritive values per serving: *cal 117, cho 8 gm, pro 14 gm, fat 3 gm, Na 1,039 mg*
Food exchanges per serving: *2 lean meat and 1/2 bread*
Low sodium diets: *Use low-sodium beef broth and meat cooked without salt.*
Low cholesterol diets: *Remove all visible fat from the meat.*
Yield: *1 quart, 4 servings*

Corn Soup

I live in Iowa, after all, and I couldn't do a cookbook without a recipe for corn soup.

2 Tablespoons (1/4 stick) margarine
2 Tablespoons shredded carrots
2 Tablespoons chopped fresh or frozen green peppers
3 Tablespoons all-purpose flour
1 1/4 cups fat free chicken broth
1 cup 2% milk
1 3/4 cups (16-ounce can) cream-style corn
1/8 teaspoon celery salt
1/4 teaspoon salt
1/8 teaspoon white pepper

Melt margarine in a 2- to 3-quart saucepan, add carrots and peppers and cook over moderate heat, stirring frequently, until vegetables are soft but not browned. Add flour to the vegetables and cook and stir until vegetables are covered with flour. Add broth and milk to the vegetables and cook, stirring frequently, over moderate heat until thickened and smooth. Add corn, celery salt, salt and pepper to the sauce. Cook and stir until well blended and hot enough to serve, using 1 cup soup per serving.

Nutritive values per serving: *cal 190, cho 28 gm, pro 5 gm, fat 8 gm, Na 1,078mg*

Food exchanges per serving: *1 bread, 2 vegetable and 1 fat*

Low-sodium diets: *Omit salt. Use low-sodium broth, salt-free margarine and celery seed instead of celery salt.*

Low-cholesterol diets: *Use skim milk instead of 2% milk.*

Yield: *1 quart, 4 servings*

Cream of Vegetable Soup

This is a basic soup which can be used with many different vegetables. The liquid in which the vegetables have been cooked can also be used as part of the liquid without any change in the food exchanges. Fresh or frozen vegetables will give you a much better soup although canned vegetables may also be used, if desired.

1 1/2 cups finely chopped, cooked asparagus, broccoli, carrots, cauliflower, celery, mushrooms, onions, yellow or green string beans or a combination of any of them.
3 1/2 cups fat-free chicken broth
1/4 cup all-purpose flour
1/4 cup instant dry milk
2 Tablespoons melted margarine
salt to taste
a sprinkle of pepper (optional)

Cook vegetables, drain well and chop into small pieces suitable for soup. Refrigerate vegetables if they are not to be used within 30 minutes. Place broth in a saucepan and bring to a simmer over moderate heat. Place flour, dry milk and melted margarine in a small bowl and mix well to form coarse crumbs. Stir the flour mixture all at once into the simmering broth, using a wire whip. (This recipe will not work using a spoon. If you want to use a spoon, add the flour mixture to the cold broth and cook and stir over moderate heat to form a sauce.) Cook and stir over moderate heat until mixture is smooth and the starchy taste is gone. Add the vegetables to the sauce and reheat to serving temperature. Taste for seasoning and add salt, if necessary, along with the pepper. (Nutritive values are based on the use of commercial broth, with no added salt.) Serve hot, using 1 cup per serving.

Nutritive values per serving: *cal 121, cho 12 gm, pro 5 gm, fat 6 gm, Na 1,099 mg. This recipe can be a good source of fiber.*
Food exchanges per serving: *1 skim milk and 1 fat*
Low-sodium diets: *Use fresh or frozen vegetables cooked without salt, low-sodium broth and salt-free margarine. Do not add any salt to the soup.*
Low-cholesterol diets: *May be used as written.*
Yield: *1 quart, 4 servings*

Minestrone Soup

I think Chuck must get a little tired of this soup along about spring. I like it so much that I prepare it at least a couple of times every month during the winter. (It is really just a good vegetable-beef soup with Italian seasoning.) Minestrone varies from one part of Italy to another, but it almost always contains some form of dried beans and pasta of some sort. I include the beans in mine because of their fiber but I don't include the pasta because I'd rather have crackers with my soup. If you want spaghetti or noodles in your soup, remember that 1/2 cup pasta or noodles is 1 bread exchange, and add however much you want to your bowl of soup when you are ready to eat it.

1 quart hot fat-free beef broth
1/2 cup chopped onions
1/4 cup chopped fresh or frozen green peppers
1/2 cup chopped carrots
1/4 cup chopped celery
1 cup cooked, drained navy or great northern beans
1 teaspoon salt
1 cup chopped canned tomatoes with juice
1 cup cubed fresh white potatoes
1 cup finely shredded cabbage
1 cup (6 ounces) cooked, diced beef with fat and gristle removed
1 to 2 teaspoons Italian seasoning
Sprinkle of pepper

Place beef broth, onions, green peppers, carrots, celery, beans and salt in a 3-quart saucepan, cover and simmer for 10 minutes. Add tomatoes, potatoes and cabbage, cover and simmer another 15 minutes. Add beef and seasonings and simmer another 5 minutes. Check for seasoning and add a sprinkle of pepper and salt, if necessary. (The amount of salt necessary will depend upon the saltiness of the broth.) Serve hot, using 1 cup soup per serving.

Nutritive values per serving:
With beans: *cal 131, cho 16 gm, pro 12 gm, fat 2 gm, Na 857 mg. This recipe is a good source of fiber.*
Without beans: *cal 100, cho 11 gm, pro 10 gm, fat 2 gm, Na 754 mg. This recipe is a good source of fiber.*

Food exchanges per serving:
With beans: *1 bread and 1 1/2 lean meat*
Without beans: *2 vegetable, and 1 lean meat*

Low-sodium diets: *Do not add salt; use salt-free broth.*

Low-cholesterol diets: *May be used as written.*

Yield: *1 1/2 quarts with beans, 6 servings; 1 1/4 quarts without beans, 6 servings*

Mushroom Tomato Soup

This soup is a lovely pale pink with a subtle mushroom and tomato flavor. It is good hot on a cold day or chilled in the summertime.

1 Tablespoon margarine
1/4 cup finely chopped onions
1/2 cup chopped mushrooms
3 Tablespoons all-purpose flour
1 1/2 cups fat-free chicken broth
1 cup 2% milk
1/2 cup tomato sauce
1/8 teaspoon sweet basil
1/8 teaspoon salt
sprinkle of pepper

Melt margarine in a 1 1/2- to 2-quart saucepan over low heat. Add onions and mushrooms and cook and stir over moderate heat until the onions are soft but not browned. Add flour to the vegetables and cook and stir over moderate heat until the vegetables are coated with flour. Add broth and milk to the vegetables. Mix well and then add tomato sauce, basil, salt and pepper. Cook over moderate heat, stirring frequently, until the soup begins to simmer. Cook and stir until thickened and smooth. Use 1 cup per serving and serve hot or chilled according to the weather.

Nutritive values per serving: *cal 128, cho 15 gm, pro 5 gm, fat 6 gm, Na 1,070 mg*
Food exchanges per serving: *1 bread, 1 fat*
Low-sodium diets: *Omit salt. Use salt-free margarine, low-sodium broth and tomato sauce canned without salt.*
Low-cholesterol diets: *Use skim milk instead of 2% milk and add 1 teaspoon margarine when cooking the vegetables.*
Yield: *3 cups, 3 servings*

Potato Soup

Everybody has a security blanket, and this is my sister's. This is what our mother made for us when we were children if we didn't feel well, and it still makes both of us feel loved and cherished.

1/4 cup finely chopped onions
1 Tablespoon finely chopped celery
1 1/2 cups water
1/2 cup diced fresh potatoes
1/2 cup water
2 Tablespoons all-purpose flour
1/4 teaspoon salt
1 teaspoon margarine
1 cup 2% milk
sprinkle of pepper (optional)

Combine onions, celery and 1 1/2 cups water in a small saucepan. Cover and simmer for 10 minutes. Add potatoes, cover and simmer for 15 to 20 minutes or until the potatoes are tender. Combine 1/2 cup water, flour and salt and stir to make a smooth paste. Add to the soup and cook and stir until the soup is thickened and the starchy taste is gone. Add margarine, milk and pepper to the soup. Reheat to serving temperature and serve hot, using 1/2 of the soup, about 1 cup, per serving.

Nutritive values per serving: *cal 151, cho 21 gm, pro 7 gm, fat 5 gm, Na 360 mg*
Food exchanges per serving: *1 skim milk, 1/2 bread and 1/2 fat*
Low-sodium diets: *Omit salt. Use salt-free margarine.*
Low-cholesterol diets: *Use skim milk and 2 teaspoons margarine.*
Yield: *about 2 cups, 2 servings*

Chapter 7

ENTRÉES

The complete protein found in meat, fish and poultry is very important to us. We don't need the one-pound steaks and twelve-ounce cuts of rare roast beef common in our grandparents' day, but we do need an adequate supply of protein.

Now that we have a high complex carbohydrate diet—and I'm very happy about it—we need to compensate for the extra calories in the added carbohydrate by cutting down on our fat intake. Fortunately, the beef and pork growers have seen the light and have been breeding cattle and hogs with a lower percentage of fat so that we can get meat which is tender and good and still keep our fat intake as low as possible. Fish and poultry are also low in fat and doctors say we should have them several times a week.

We need to be selective in our choice of meats to get the best possible flavor with the lowest amount of fat. I can see an occasional slice of bacon for flavor, but bacon and an egg every morning for breakfast just doesn't fit into the low-cholesterol diet that I think most diabetics should follow. I firmly believe that ground meat should be browned and the fat discarded, all possible fat should be trimmed from meat before it is cooked, and roasts, chicken and turkey should be cooked on a rack so that all of the fat will go to the bottom of the pan where it can be discarded. These rules may cause a little bit more work in the beginning but eventually they become such a habit that you do them without thinking about it.

Almost everyone knows how to cook a roast, grill a steak or broil chicken or fish, simmer meat and chill it to remove the fat. We have been living on that kind of meat for years. If you aren't knowledgeable about those recipes, there are many good cookbooks which can give you that information in great detail.

I have chosen, in this book, to give you recipes for casseroles and other recipes which contain complex carbohydrates. Most of us aren't accustomed to that sort of recipe, because it is only recently that we have been able to think in terms of actually adding carbohydrates to foods—and I love doing it. I'm perfectly willing to give up a slice of bread—even though I love bread—in order to have a good casserole with some rice, noodles or macaroni in it.

If you would like to make your own casserole for yourself or someone else, you can analyze your recipe in one of two ways. You can get very technical and analyze the recipe according to complete nutritional information, as I do for all recipes I publish, or you could do it the simpler way by taking information from the food packages or from the food exchange lists in Chapter 3.

When I started analyzing recipes for diabetic diets, I drew up the following chart which you might also find useful.

Recipe Analysis

Name of Recipe:__________________ Date tested:_________

Source of Recipe:______________________________

Type and Number of Pans Used:____________________

Temperature:_____ Baking or Cooking Time:_____

No. of Servings:_____

Size of Servings:__________ Comments:_______________

Ingredients	Amount	Cal	Cho gm	Pro gm	Fat gm	Na mg

Total nutritive values						
Divided by the total no. of portions						
Rounded to the nearest number						
Number of food exchanges equal to nutritive value						

If you want to use this chart to prepare your own casserole of tunafish, noodles and mushrooms, you would first enter on the chart all of the ingredients that you would use for the casserole:

1 1/2 cups cooked macaroni
10 3/4-ounce can Campbells condensed cream of mushroom soup
water
6 1/2-ounce can Star-Kist chunk tuna packed in spring water
4 1/2-ounce can Green Giant mushrooms

You could follow the nutritive information on the macaroni package, but it gets a little complicated, so you could also use the information from the listing of food exchanges in Chapter 3. There you will find that 1/2 cup of cooked macaroni is 1 bread exchange. You will also find that a bread exchange is 80 calories, 15 grams of carbohydrate (carb) and 3 grams of protein (pro), so you multiply these values by 3 for the 3 bread exchanges and enter the results on your chart.

Next you look at the label on the soup can and find that the can provides 2 3/4 servings of soup. The nutritive values for each serving are on the can, so to find the total value of the soup, you multiply the values for each serving by 2 3/4 or 2.75. (I have a calculator which comes in very handy.)

100 calories × 2.75 = 275 calories
1 gram of protein × 2.75 = 2.75 or 2.8 grams of protein
9 grams of carbohydrate × 2.75 = 24.75 or 24.8 grams of carbohydrate
7 grams of fat × 2.75 = 19.25 or 19.3 grams of fat
825 mg. of Na (sodium) × 2.75 = 2,268.75 or 2.269 mg. of sodium

Water doesn't have any food value, so you don't have to worry about it. Some people would use milk to thin the soup for the casserole, but milk would provide more carbohydrate and I prefer the taste of water, so I use water. If you wanted to use milk you would look it up in Chapter 3 and use the values for 1/2 cup skim milk (6 grams of carbohydrate and 4 grams of protein).

You know that a 6 1/2-ounce can of tunafish packed in water will yield 6 1/2 ounces of drained tunafish, so you could use 6 1/2 times the values for 1 meat exchange which would be 6 1/2 × 7 grams of protein and 3 grams of fat (for a lean meat exchange), but since the can has the nutritive values on it for the drained tunafish, I would prefer to use that. Exchanges are necessarily rounded for ease of use, while information on the can is more accurate. As you read the information on the can (with a magnifying glass) you see that the can has 3.3 servings of 2 ounces each so you multiply the values given for the carbohydrate, protein, fat and sodium on the can by 3.3 and enter those figures also on the chart.

The mushrooms that I'm using for this recipe are in a 4 1/2-ounce jar which the label says is 2 1/4 2-ounce servings so you would again multiply the nutritive information on the jar for 1 serving by 2.25 to get the total nutritive values of the mushrooms and then enter those on your chart.

Now you have all of the ingredients that go into the casserole so you add up those ingredients to get the total nutritive values of the casserole. When you have the total nutritive values, you divide that by the number of servings to get the nutritive values for each serving.

Recipe Analysis

Name of Recipe: Tuna, Noodle & Mushroom Date Tested: 6/16
Source of Recipe: My own favorite recipe
Type & Number of Pans: 1 1 1/2 qt Corning Ware casserole
Temperature: 350°F Baking or Cooking Time: 25-30 min
No. of Servings 4
Size of Servings: About 1 cup Comments: Chuck likes it. I doubled it and took it to club and they liked it very much.

Ingredients	Amount	Cal	Cho gm	Pro gm	Fat gm	Na mg
Cooked macaroni	1 1/2 cups	240	45.0	9.0		
Mushroom soup	10 3/4 ounce	275.	24.8	2.8	19.3	2,269
Tunafish	6 1/2 ounces	198	3.0	42.9	3.0	1,089
Mushrooms	4 1/2 ounces	32	4.5	2.3		585
Total nutritive values		745	77.3	57.0	22.3	3,943

Divided by the total no. of portions 4	186.3	19.3	14.3	5.6	985.8
Rounded to the nearest number	186	19	14	6	986
Number of food exchanges equal to nutritive value					
1 bread	80	15	3		
2 lean meat	110		14	6	
Total	190	15	17	6	

Note: Exchanges are never exact. You try to come as close to the total as possible and then use that number of exchanges.

Sometimes you don't know the number of servings or the yield of the recipe until after it is cooked. In that case, you have to measure the actual yield so that you know how much of the casserole will constitute a serving. At other times, when you do the analysis, you will realize that you can't afford to use some of the ingredients which have too high a content of carbohydrate or fat and you will have to cut down on them. I have found that it is amazing how far I can cut down on fat and still get a good cream sauce, and you can generally cut the sugar content of baked goods by 2/3 or 3/4 and still get good results.

If you are interested in lowering the sodium content of your diet, you are better off using the information on the cans which include sodium information because the food exchanges do not include sodium content. If you want to add salt to a casserole, include 2.132 mg. of salt per teaspoon of salt. And when you see the sodium content of commercial broths and bouillons, you will be in favor of using the low-sodium broths or making your own. Canned soups are high in sodium when they are used in casseroles, but fortunately there are quite a few low-sodium canned soups available now which fit well into casseroles.

Baked Meatballs

These meatballs are excellent with spaghetti and also good served with noodles without the Italian seasoning.

2 eggs
1/2 cup water
1 teaspoon salt
Sprinkle of pepper
1 teaspoon Italian seasoning
1/2 cup finely chopped onions
3 slices commercial whole wheat bread cut into 1-inch chunks
2 pounds lean ground beef

Place eggs, water, salt, pepper, Italian seasoning, onions and bread in mixer bowl and mix until the bread is broken up into small bits. Add the ground beef and mix at medium speed only to blend. Do not overmix. Form meat balls using a level No. 16 dipper (1/4 cup) of the meat mixture for each ball. Place the balls in a shallow pan and bake at 350°F for 30 minutes, or until browned and firm. Remove the meatballs from the pan and serve hot, using 2 meatballs per serving.

Nutritive values per serving: *cal 223, cho 5 gm, pro 23 gm, fat 6 gm, Na 288 mg*
Food exchanges per serving: *1/3 bread and 3 lean meat*
Low-sodium diets: *Omit salt.*
Low-cholesterol diets: *Omit eggs. Use 3 egg whites.*
Yield: *18 meatballs, 9 servings*

Baked Sandwiches

It is handy to have a batch of these in the freezer to serve for lunch on a day when you are too busy to cook or to take along on an unexpected picnic. They are best if allowed to defrost in the refrigerator but they can defrost on the way to a picnic or in the microwave if you want them in a hurry.

1 1/4 cups water at 110 to 115°F
1 package (2 1/4 teaspoons) quick-rise yeast
2 cups all-purpose flour
1 teaspoon salt
1 egg
2 Tablespoons vegetable oil
1 1/2 cups graham flour
1 1/2 pounds lean ground beef
1/2 cup chopped onions
1 cup tomato sauce
1/4 cup catsup
1 teaspoon garlic salt
1/2 teaspoon leaf oregano
Sprinkle of pepper

Combine water and yeast in mixer bowl and let stand for 5 minutes. Add all-purpose flour and mix at medium speed, using a dough hook, for 4 minutes. Add salt, egg, vegetable oil and graham flour and mix at medium speed for another 4 minutes. Turn the dough out onto a lightly floured board and knead a few times, form into a ball and place in a well-greased mixing bowl. Turn the ball over to grease the top, cover with a cloth and let stand at room temperature to rise until doubled in volume.

While the dough is rising, cook the meat and onions in the fat from the meat over medium heat, stirring frequently, until the onions are soft and the meat is browned and well separated. Drain the meat and onion mixture, discard the fat and juice and return meat and onions to the pan. Add tomato sauce, catsup, garlic salt, oregano and pepper and cook and stir over medium heat until the meat is dry with no noticeable liquid. Set meat mixture aside to cool until dough is ready.

After the dough has doubled in volume, transfer it to a lightly floured working surface. Knead lightly. Form into a roll and cut into 12 equal portions. Form each portion into a little ball, cover with a cloth and let rest for 10 minutes.

Roll each ball out to form a circle 5 to 6 inches across. Put 1/12 (about 1/4 cup) of the meat mixture in the center of the circle. Pull the dough up around the filling and press together at the top. Place on a well greased cookie sheet, cover with a cloth and let stand about 30 to 40 minutes at room temperature or until doubled in volume. Bake at 350°F for 40 to 45 minutes or until lightly browned and firm. Serve hot, using 1 sandwich per serving, or refrigerate or freeze to be used later.

Nutritive values per serving: *cal 293, cho 27 gm, pro 21 gm, fat 9 gm, Na 574 mg*

Food exchanges per serving: *2 bread and 2 lean meat*

Low-sodium diets: *Omit salt and garlic salt. Use low-sodium tomato sauce and catsup and 1/4 teaspoon powdered garlic.*

Low-cholesterol diets: *Omit egg. Use 2 egg whites or 1/4 cup liquid egg substitute.*

Yield: *12 sandwiches, 12 servings*

Beans and Beef

I took this casserole along to a birthday party for our neighbor Butch Franks. His sister and father-in-law are diabetic also, and everyone liked it enough to ask for the recipe, which I consider the ultimate compliment.

1 Tablespoon vegetable oil
1 cup chopped onions
1 cup chopped fresh green peppers
12 ounces lean ground beef
1 3/4 cups (15-ounce can) drained butter beans
1 3/4 cups (15-ounce can) drained pinto beans
1 teaspoon garlic salt
1/8 teaspoon red pepper
2 Tablespoons soy sauce
1 cup tomato sauce

Heat a 2-quart saucepan over moderate heat for 1/2 minute, add the oil and swirl it around the bottom of the pan. Place the onions and green peppers in the pan and cook and stir over moderate heat until the onions are soft. Add meat to the vegetables and cook and stir until the meat is well browned and broken apart. Drain the meat and vegetable mixture well and then return to the saucepan along with the beans, garlic salt, red pepper, soy sauce and tomato sauce. Heat, stirring frequently, to serving temperature and serve hot, using 3/4 cup per serving.

Note: You can put the mixture in a casserole in the oven at 350°F for 20 to 30 minutes to reheat and thicken instead of reheating it on top of the stove.

Nutritive values per serving: *cal 249, cho 19 gm, pro 18 gm, fat 7 gm, Na 921 mg. This recipe is a good source of fiber.*

Food exchanges per serving: *1 bread, 1 vegetable and 2 lean meat*

Low-sodium diets: *Omit garlic salt and soy sauce. Use beans and tomato sauce cooked without salt and 1/4 teaspoon powdered garlic.*

Low-cholesterol diets: *May be used as written.*

Yield: *1 1/2 quarts, 8 servings*

Hamburger with Brown Rice

12 ounces lean ground beef
1/3 cup brown rice
1 4-ounce can sliced mushrooms
3/4 cup hot fat-free beef broth
1/2 cup chopped onions
2 Tablespoons soy sauce
1/2 teaspoon salt
1/8 teaspoon pepper

Cook and stir ground beef in a heavy frying pan over medium heat until the meat is broken up and well browned. Drain well and then put the meat in a crockpot that has been preheated on high. Add rice, mushrooms with their juice, beef broth, onions, soy sauce, salt and pepper. Cook, stirring occasionally, on high in the crockpot about 2 hours or until the rice is tender. Serve hot, using 3/4 cup per serving.

Nutritive values per serving: *cal 237, cho 15 gm, pro 20 gm, fat 9 gm, Na 990 mg*
Food exchanges per serving: *1 bread and 3 lean meat*
Low-sodium diets: *Omit salt and soy sauce. Season with 1/2 teaspoon Italian seasoning or 1/2 teaspoon chili seasoning.*
Low-cholesterol diets: *May be used as written.*
Yield: *3 cups, 4 servings*

Pasticchio ✓

I've taken this Greek casserole to several pot luck dinners and everyone seems to like it very much. If you want it spicier, double the pepper and add 1/4 teaspoon nutmeg to the meat mixture.

1 1/2 cups (6 ounces) elbow macaroni
1/4 cup grated Parmesan cheese
1/2 cup 2% milk
1 beaten egg
3/4 pound lean ground beef
1/2 cup chopped onions
1 cup canned tomato sauce
1/2 teaspoon salt
1/2 teaspoon cinnamon
1/8 teaspoon pepper
1 Tablespoon melted margarine
3 Tablespoons all-purpose flour
1/3 cup instant dry milk
1/4 teaspoon salt
1 1/2 cups boiling water
1 beaten egg
1/4 cup grated Parmesan cheese

Cook macaroni according to directions on the package and drain well. While noodles are still hot, mix together 1/4 cup grated Parmesan cheese, 1/2 cup milk and 1 beaten egg and add to noodles. Set aside.

Cook and stir meat and onions together in a frying pan over medium heat until onions are soft and meat is browned and broken into small pieces. Drain well. Return the drained meat and onions to the frying pan, add the tomato sauce, salt, cinnamon and pepper. Mix well and set aside.

Stir the melted margarine, flour, dry milk and salt together to blend well, stir into the boiling water and cook, using a whip, until thickened and smooth. (It is important to use a whip: if you don't, add the flour mixture to cool water and then cook and stir over moderate heat until thickened and smooth.) Mix the beaten egg and 1/4 cup grated Parmesan cheese together and stir the hot sauce into it. Spread 1/2 of the macaroni evenly in the bottom of a greased 9″

square baking pan. Spread the meat mixture evenly over the macaroni and then top with the remaining macaroni. Spread the sauce evenly over the top of the macaroni and bake at 350°F for about 45 minutes, until lightly browned. Cut the casserole into 9 equal portions and serve hot, using 1 portion per serving.

Nutritive values per serving: *cal 232, cho 20 gm, pro 18 gm, fat 8 gm, Na 455 mg*

Food exchanges per serving: *1 bread, 1 vegetable, 2 lean meat*

Low-sodium diets: *Omit salt. Use low sodium tomato sauce and fat-free margarine.*

Low-cholesterol diets: *Omit eggs. Use 1/4 cup liquid egg substitute for each egg.*

Yield: *1 9-inch casserole, 9 servings*

Tomato–Meat Sauce for Spaghetti

This is a rather mild sauce. If you like a spicier sauce, you can increase the amount of spice or use your own favorite spices without any change in the food exchange values.

1 Tablespoon vegetable oil
1 cup chopped onions
1/4 cup chopped fresh green peppers
1/4 cup chopped celery
12 ounces lean ground beef
1 6-ounce can tomato paste
1 Tablespoon sugar
1 16-ounce can tomatoes
2 15-ounce cans tomato sauce
2 cups double strength fat-free chicken broth
1/2 teaspoon garlic powder
Sprinkle of pepper
1 teaspoon Italian seasoning

Preheat a heavy 4-quart saucepan on medium heat for 15 seconds, swirl oil around the bottom of the pan, add onions, green peppers and celery and cook and stir over medium heat until the onions are soft but not browned. Add beef to the vegetables and cook and stir over medium heat until the meat is well browned and broken up. Drain the meat and vegetables well, discarding the fat and liquid. Wash the pan well with hot water. Return the meat and vegetables to the pan. Add tomato paste, sugar, tomatoes, tomato sauce and broth to the meat mixture and simmer, stirring frequently, over low heat for 30 minutes. Add garlic, pepper and Italian seasoning to the sauce and continue to simmer, stirring frequently, for another 30 minutes, or until the sauce is thickened. (There should be no liquid when you put a Tablespoonful of the sauce on a saucer.) Taste for seasoning and add more, if desired, or use your own favorite seasoning combination. Serve the sauce hot, using 1/2 cup of sauce per serving, over hot, well-drained spaghetti or noodles, or use the sauce for lasagna or other recipes which require a tomato-meat sauce.

Nutritive values per serving:
1/2 cup: *cal 92, cho 10 gm, pro 7 gm, fat 3 gm, Na 636 mg. This recipe is a good source of fiber.*
1 cup: *cal 184, cho 20 gm, pro 14 gm, fat 6 gm, Na 1,272 mg*

Food exchanges per serving:
1/2 cup: *2 vegetable and 1/2 medium-fat meat*
1 cup: *1 bread, 1 vegetable and 1 medium-fat meat*

Low-sodium diets: *Use low-sodium canned tomato paste, tomato sauce, tomatoes and chicken broth.*

Low-cholesterol diets: *May be used as written.*

Yield: *7 cups—14 1/2-cup or 7 1-cup servings*

Brown Gravy

This is the time to use those drippings that you have saved from roasts, because the flavor of the gravy will depend upon the flavor of the broth or drippings.

3 Tablespoons all-purpose flour
1 Tablespoon melted margarine
2 1/4 cups fat-free broth or drippings
Sprinkle of pepper
1/2 teaspoon Kitchen Bouquet (optional)

Stir flour and margarine together until smooth. Place broth or drippings in small saucepan, bring to a boil and then add the flour mixture, stirring constantly with a wire whip. (This will not work with a spoon. If you don't have a whip, add the flour mixture to cold drippings or broth and stir and cook over medium heat until thickened.) Cook and stir over medium heat until smooth and thick. Add pepper and Kitchen Bouquet, mix and serve hot, using 1/4 cup per serving.

Nutritive values per serving: *cal 26, cho 2 gm, pro 1 gm, fat 2 gm, Na variable*
Food exchanges per serving: *1/4 cup may be considered free.*
Low-sodium diets: *Use low-sodium broth or drippings and salt-free margarine. Omit Kitchen Bouquet.*
Low-cholesterol diets: *May be used as written.*
Yield: *2 cups, 8 servings*

Stir-Fried Pork and Vegetables

1 1/2 cups fat-free chicken broth
2 Tablespoons cornstarch
2 Tablespoons teriyaki sauce
1 Tablespoon vegetable oil
1 cup thinly sliced carrots
1 cup celery cut into thin diagonal slices
1/2 cup chopped onions
1/2 cup (4 ounces) canned sliced mushrooms, drained
1 Tablespoon vegetable oil
1 pound boneless fresh ham, cut into very thin slices
1 4-ounce can drained and thinly sliced Chinese chestnuts (water chestnuts)

Combine chicken broth, cornstarch and teriyaki sauce, mix until smooth and set aside.

Preheat a large frying pan over medium heat for 1/2 minute. (A frying pan with a Silverstone or other hard finish works best.) Swirl 1 Tablespoon vegetable oil around the bottom of the pan and then add carrots, celery, onions and mushrooms and cook and stir over high heat for 5 to 8 minutes or until tender but still crisp. Remove the vegetables with a slotted spoon and set aside. Swirl 1 Tablespoon vegetable oil in the frying pan, add the pork and cook and stir over high heat about 5 minutes or until all traces of pink are gone from the pork. Add the chicken broth mixture to the pork and cook and stir over medium heat until thickened and smooth. Add the vegetable mixture to the pork along with the Chinese chestnuts and reheat to serving temperature. Serve hot, using 3/4 cup pork and vegetables per serving.

Nutritive values per serving: *cal 194, cho 8 gm, pro 17 gm, fat 10 gm, Na 851 mg. This recipe is a good source of fiber.*

Food exchanges per serving: *2 vegetable and 2 medium-fat meat*

Low-sodium diets: *Omit teriyaki sauce and use low-sodium broth.*

Low-cholesterol diets: *May be used as written.*

Yield: *1 quart, 6 servings*

Chicken Lasagna

I'm not Italian, but my husband is, and our friends seem to expect us to serve Italian food frequently. This is one of our party favorites which is easy to prepare and can be made and frozen several days, or even longer, before a party. I like to defrost it in the refrigerator before I cook it, but you can bake it directly from the freezer if you add about 30 minutes to the baking time.

1 pound part skim milk ricotta cheese
3 medium eggs
2 Tablespoons grated Parmesan cheese
2 Tablespoons chopped parsley
1/2 teaspoon garlic powder
7 ounces lasagna noodles
1/2 cup chopped canned mushrooms
1 10 3/4 ounce can condensed cream of chicken soup
1 cup double strength fat-free chicken broth
1 cup (6 ounces) diced cooked chicken with fat and skin removed
8 ounces grated low-fat mozzarella cheese
2 Tablespoons grated Parmesan cheese
1 teaspoon leaf oregano

Combine ricotta cheese, eggs, 2 Tablespoons Parmesan cheese, parsley and garlic powder in a small bowl. Mix lightly but well and set aside. The mixture should be refrigerated if it is not to be used within the hour but should be brought back to room temperature before it is used.

Cook lasagna noodles according to directions on the package. Drain well. Run cold water over the noodles and drain well before they are used. (They may be allowed to stand in cold water for a time if they are cooked before the lasagna is prepared.)

Combine mushrooms, chicken soup and double strength chicken broth and stir to blend well to form a sauce.

Layer the lasagna in a 9″ square pan in the following order:

1. 3/4 cup sauce in the bottom of the pan;
2. 1/3 of the noodles laid flat on the sauce;
3. 1/2 of the ricotta cheese mixture spread evenly over the noodles;
4. 1/2 of the grated mozzarella cheese sprinkled evenly over the cheese;
5. 3/4 cup sauce;
6. 1/3 of the noodles;
7. the remainder of the ricotta cheese filling;
8. the remainder of the mozzarella cheese;
9. 3/4 cup of the sauce;
10. the remainder of the noodles;
11. the remainder of the sauce;
12. 2 Tablespoons of Parmesan cheese sprinkled evenly over the sauce;
13. Leaf oregano sprinkled evenly over the top.

Bake at 350°F 45 minutes to 1 hour, or until the top is lightly browned and bubbling. Remove from oven and let stand 15 to 20 minutes to firm up before cutting the lasagna into 9 equal portions. Use 1 portion per serving.

Variation:

Vegetable Lasagna—Omit chicken and chicken soup. Substitute 1 10 3/4-ounce can condensed cream of mushroom soup and 2 cups cooked, diced vegetables such as broccoli, onions, carrots, green or yellow string beans or a mixture of these and other vegetables found in the vegetable exchange list. (One portion yields 1 bread, 1 milk, 1 medium-fat meat and 2 fat exchanges.)

Nutritive values per serving: *cho 23 gm, pro 27 gm, fat 15 gm, Na 807 mg*

Food exchanges per serving: *1 1/2 bread and 3 medium-fat meat*

Low-sodium diets: *Use low-sodium soups and chicken broth.*

Low-cholesterol diets: *Omit eggs. Use 3/4 cup liquid egg substitute, or 3 large egg whites.*

Yield: *1 9" square pan, 9 servings*

Pineapple Chicken

Gail Olson of Volga City, Iowa, with whom I've had some very interesting conversations about food preparation, gave me this recipe, which we enjoy. Her recipe included brown sugar, but I find we like it with the brown sugar substitute also.

1 Tablespoon vegetable oil
1 cup fresh green peppers, julienned
1 cup diagonally sliced celery
1/2 cup chopped onions
1 1/2 cups fat-free chicken broth
3 Tablespoons cornstarch
1/4 cup vinegar
1/4 cup soy sauce
1 1/4 teaspoons Sweet 'n Low brown sugar substitute
1 cup pineapple chunks, canned without sugar, drained well
1 cup (6 ounces) cooked diced chicken with fat and gristle removed
1 medium sized fresh tomato, cut into wedges

Preheat a 2-quart saucepan over medium heat for 1/2 minute, swirl the oil around the bottom of the pan and then add the green peppers, celery and onions. Cook, stirring frequently, over medium heat until the vegetables are tender but crisp (about 10 minutes). Set aside in the pan.

Combine chicken broth, cornstarch, vinegar and soy sauce in a small saucepan, stir to a smooth paste and then cook and stir over medium heat until smooth and thickened. Remove sauce from the heat, stir the brown sugar substitute into the sauce and then add the sauce, pineapple and chicken to the vegetable mixture. Reheat over medium heat, stirring lightly, add the tomatoes and heat only until the tomato is slightly warmed. Serve hot, using 3/4 cup of the pineapple chicken per serving.

Nutritive values per serving: *cal 220, cho 22 gm, pro 23 gm, fat 15 gm, Na 1,957 mg. This recipe is a good source of fiber.*

Food exchanges per serving: *1 fruit, 1 vegetable and 3 medium-fat meat*

Low-sodium diets: *Use low-sodium broth and omit the soy sauce.*

Low-cholesterol diets: *May be used as written.*

Yield: *3 cups, 4 servings*

Chili with Turkey

1 Tablespoon vegetable oil
1/2 cup chopped onions
1 pound ground raw turkey
1 16-ounce can chopped tomatoes
1 15-ounce can tomato sauce
1 cup fat-free chicken broth
1 Tablespoon chili powder
1 teaspoon paprika
1 teaspoon garlic salt
1/8 teaspoon pepper (optional)
1/4 teaspoon oregano
1/4 teaspoon cumin
1 16-ounce can pinto beans

Preheat heavy 3-quart saucepan over medium heat for 1/2 minute. Swirl oil in the bottom of the pan, add onions and cook and stir until onions are soft but not browned. Add turkey to onions and cook, stirring frequently, until turkey is broken up and no pink remains. Drain turkey well, discarding any liquid and fat. Return turkey to the saucepan and add tomatoes, tomato sauce, broth, chili powder, paprika, garlic salt, pepper, oregano and cumin. Simmer, uncovered, over very low heat, stirring occasionally, for 1 hour. Add pinto beans and their liquid and cook, stirring occasionally, for another 15 minutes. Serve hot, using 1 cup chili per serving.

Note: More or less chili powder may be used without changing the food exchanges.

Nutritive values per serving: *cal 329, cho 33 gm, pro 22 gm, fat 8 gm, Na 893 mg. This recipe is a good source of fiber.*

Food exchanges per serving: *2 bread, 1 vegetable, 2 lean meat*

Low-sodium diets: *Omit garlic salt. Use 1/4 teaspoon garlic. Use low-sodium broth and tomatoes and tomato sauce canned without salt.*

Low-cholesterol diets: *May be used as written.*

Yield: *1 1/2 quarts, 6 servings*

Pot Roasted Turkey Legs

Turkey legs
sage
salt and pepper
1/2 cup water
potatoes
onions
carrots
salt and pepper to taste

This is a method more than a recipe since the amounts you use will depend upon how many you are serving and whether you want to have turkey to freeze for future casseroles. I generally roast about 6 legs at a time which is sufficient for dinner with quite a bit left to freeze for future use.

Ask your butcher to cut the turkey legs crosswise for you, dividing each one of them into three pieces: a bony part at the bottom which is saved for broth-making and two equal portions from the fleshy part of the leg. Place the fleshy parts of the legs in an uncovered roaster and bake at 375°F for 1 hour. Sprinkle the legs with sage, salt and pepper, add water to the roaster, cover and bake at 325°F for 1 hour. Remove the roaster from the oven, add the potatoes, onions and carrots, sprinkle them with salt and pepper, cover the roaster and roast for another hour or until the vegetables are tender. (Those troublesome tendons in the turkey legs which cause so much trouble are very easy to remove after the meat is tender.) Serve the turkey and vegetables, counting exchanges for the portion used. After the unused turkey is cool enough to handle, remove the meat from the bones and freeze in portions to use for future casseroles.

Nutritive values per serving: *Nutritive values will depend upon the amounts used.*

Food exchanges per serving: *Calculate the exchanges used according to the amounts used.*

Low-sodium diets: *Omit salt.*

Low-cholesterol diets: *May be used as written.*

Yield: *Depends upon the amount prepared.*

Turkey Loaf

6 Saltine crackers
1 egg
1 crushed chicken bouillon cube
1/2 teaspoon salt
1/4 teaspoon sage, thyme or poultry seasoning
sprinkle of pepper
1 pound ground raw turkey

Crush crackers and put them into a mixer bowl along with the egg, bouillon cube, salt, sage, thyme or poultry seasoning and pepper. Mix at low speed 1/2 minute to blend well. Add turkey to egg mixture and mix at medium speed only until turkey is blended with the other ingredients. Do not overmix. Place turkey mixture in an 8-inch square baking pan. Form turkey mixture into a loaf about 4 by 7 1/2 inches and bake, uncovered, at 325°F for 1 1/4 to 1 1/2 hours or until lightly browned and firm. Cut loaf into 4 equal slices and use 1 slice per serving.

Nutritive values per serving: *cal 237, cho 4 gm, pro 22 gm, fat 9 gm, Na 652 mg*

Food exchanges per serving: *3 lean meat and 1 vegetable*

Low-sodium diets: *Omit salt. Use low-sodium bouillon cube.*

Low-cholesterol diets: *Omit whole egg. Use 2 egg whites.*

Yield: *1 turkey loaf, 4 servings*

Chicken Gravy

2 1/4 cups fat-free chicken broth
3 Tablespoons all-purpose flour
1 Tablespoon margarine
1/8 teaspoon poultry seasoning or thyme
sprinkle of pepper

Combine broth and flour in a small saucepan and stir until smooth. Cook and stir over medium heat until thickened and smooth. Add margarine, poultry seasoning or thyme and pepper and cook and stir 1/2 minute longer. Serve hot, using 1/4 cup per serving.

Nutritive values per serving: *cal 26, cho 2 gm, pro 1 gm, fat 2 gm, Na 314 mg*

Food exchanges per serving: *1/4 cup may be considered free.*

Low-sodium diets: *Use low-sodium broth and salt-free margarine.*

Low-cholesterol diets: *May be served as written.*

Yield: *2 cups, 8 servings*

Baked Halibut with Paprika

1 pound boneless fillet of halibut
1/2 cup chopped onions
2 Tablespoons (1/4 stick) margarine
1/3 cup evaporated skimmed milk
1 Tablespoon paprika
1/8 teaspoon pepper
1/2 teaspoon salt

Thaw the fish if necessary. Pat dry with a paper towel and set aside.

Fry the onions in the margarine over moderate heat, stirring frequently, until the onions are golden. Spread the onions in the bottom of a shallow 1-quart casserole. Cut the fish into 4 equal portions and place on top of the onions. Dribble any margarine remaining in the frying pan over the fish. Combine the milk, paprika, pepper and salt together and pour over the fish. Bake in the uncovered casserole at 375°F, basting every 5 minutes with the sauce, for 20 to 25 minutes or until the fish flakes easily when tested with a fork. Serve the fish hot from the casserole using 1 of the fish portions plus a little of the sauce per serving.

Nutritive values per serving: *cal 189, cho 4 gm, pro 26 gm, fat 7 gm, Na 411 mg*

Food exchanges per serving: *1/3 skim milk and 3 lean meat*

Low-sodium diets: *Omit salt. Use salt-free margarine.*

Low-cholesterol diets: *May be used as written.*

Yield: *4 portions, 4 servings*

Cajun Style Codfish

This recipe always reminds me of Della Andreassen, a dietitian from Lafayette, Louisiana who gave it to me. She is a Cajun who came up north to go to school and met and married her husband, a Dane, while she was up here. They eventually went back to Louisiana, which he loved almost as much as she did.

1 Tablespoon vegetable oil
1/2 cup chopped onions
1/2 cup chopped fresh green peppers
1/4 cup all-purpose flour
1 Tablespoon margarine
2 cups (16-ounce can) tomato sauce
1/4 teaspoon garlic powder
1/4 teaspoon thyme
1/8 teaspoon cayenne pepper
1/2 teaspoon salt
1 pound codfish fillets cut into 4-ounce portions

Preheat a small saucepan, swirl the vegetable oil in the bottom of the pan, add the onions and peppers and cook, stirring frequently, over medium heat until the onions are limp but not browned. Add the flour and margarine to the vegetables and cook and stir over medium heat until lightly browned. Add tomato sauce, garlic, thyme, cayenne pepper and salt and cook and stir until thickened.

Place the fillets in a 1-quart shallow casserole. Cover the fish with the hot sauce and bake uncovered at 350°F for 20 to 25 minutes or until the fish flakes easily when tested with a fork. Serve hot, using 1 of the 4-ounce portions plus some of the sauce per serving.

Nutritive values per serving: *cal 214, cho 15 gm, pro 22 gm, fat 7 gm, Na 779 mg. This recipe is a good source of fiber.*
Food exchanges per serving: *1 fruit and 3 lean meat*
Low-sodium diets: *Omit salt. Use salt free margarine and low-sodium tomato sauce.*
Low-cholesterol diets: *May be used as written.*
Yield: *4 portions, 4 servings*

Creamed Salmon and Peas

- *1 16-ounce can red salmon*
- *1 10-ounce package frozen peas*
- *2 cups fat-free chicken broth*
- *3 Tablespoons instant dry milk*
- *1/4 cup all-purpose flour*
- *1 1/2 Tablespoons margarine*
- *1/2 teaspoon salt*

Drain salmon well. Discard skin and bones and set salmon aside. Cook peas as directed on the package, drain well and set aside. Place chicken broth in a 2-quart saucepan, add dry milk and flour and stir until smooth. Add margarine, salt and pepper and cook and stir over medium heat until sauce is smooth and thick and the starchy taste is gone. Add salmon and peas to the sauce and reheat, stirring lightly, to serving temperature. Serve hot, using 3/4 cup per serving.

Nutritive values per serving: *cal 218, cho 9 gm, pro 19 gm, fat 10 gm, Na 1,066 mg. This recipe is a good source of fiber.*

Food exchanges per serving: *3/4 skim milk and 2 medium-fat meat*

Low-sodium diets: *Omit salt. Use 12 ounces fresh salmon cooked without salt and low-sodium broth.*

Low-cholesterol diets: *May be used as written.*

Yield: *1 quart, 6 servings*

Poached Fish

4-ounce fillets of codfish, halibut, haddock, etc.
water as necessary
salt as necessary

Thaw fish and cut into 4-ounce portions. Set aside, but refrigerate if it is to be more than a few minutes.

Fill shallow pan—a roaster is good—1/3 full of water, adding 1 teaspoon salt for each quart of water. (You will need a larger pan than you would think necessary, because the water may foam up as the fish is simmering.) Bring the water to a boil, add the fish, reduce the heat to low and simmer, uncovered, for 10 to 12 minutes or until the fish flakes easily. Remove the fish from the water, drain and serve hot with lemon juice (free) or tartar sauce (see p. 97), using 1 of the 4-ounce portions per serving.

Note: If you have a fish poacher, cook the fish according to the directions in the poacher and serve as directed in this recipe.

This is an excellent way to prepare fish for use in salads and casseroles.

Nutritive values per serving (based on codfish): *cal 89, cho negligible, pro 20 gm, fat negligible, Na variable.*

Food exchanges per serving: *3 lean meat*

Low-sodium diets: *Omit salt.*

Low-cholesterol diets: *May be used as written.*

Yield: *variable*

Salmon Loaf

1 16-ounce can red salmon
1/4 cup onions, chopped fine
1/4 cup celery, chopped fine
1/2 cup bread crumbs
1/2 teaspoon salt
1/2 teaspoon dill weed
sprinkle of pepper
2 eggs

Drain salmon well, put juice in mixer bowl, discard skin and bones and put salmon aside. Add onions, celery, crumbs, salt, dill, pepper and egg to salmon juice. Mix at medium speed to blend well. Add salmon to crumb mixture and mix at low speed only until blended enough to form a loaf. Spread mixture evenly in a well greased 1-quart shallow glass casserole. Bake, uncovered, at 325°F for 30 minutes. Cut into 6 equal portions and use 1 portion per serving.

Nutritive values per serving: *cal 192, cho 7 gm, pro 19 gm, fat 9 gm, Na 568 mg*

Food exchanges per serving: *1/2 skim milk and 2 medium-fat meat*

Low-sodium diets: *Omit salt. Use 12 ounces fresh salmon cooked without salt.*

Low-cholesterol diets: *Omit eggs. Use 1/2 cup liquid egg substitute.*

Yield: *1-quart casserole, 6 servings*

Tunafish, Macaroni and Broccoli

Treat this casserole gently when you are mixing it to retain as much texture as possible.

2/3 cup elbow macaroni
1 10 3/4-ounce can condensed cream of chicken soup
3/4 cup skim milk
1/2 teaspoon salt
2 cups cooked chopped broccoli
1 6 1/2-ounce can water-packed chunk tunafish
2 Tablespoons grated Parmesan cheese

Cook macaroni according to directions on the package, drain well and set aside for later use. Place soup, milk and salt in a 1 1/2-quart casserole and mix with a spoon until smooth. Lightly stir macaroni, broccoli and tunafish into the soup mixture. Sprinkle Parmesan cheese evenly over the casserole and bake at 325°F about 30 minutes or until lightly browned. Serve hot, using 1 cup of the casserole per serving.

Nutritive values per serving: *cal 204, cho 21 gm, pro 18 gm, fat 5 gm, Na 752 mg. This recipe is a good source of fiber.*
Food exchanges per serving: *1 bread, 1 vegetable and 2 lean meat*
Low-sodium diets: *Omit salt. Use low-sodium soup and tunafish.*
Low-cholesterol diets: *Omit Parmesan cheese.*
Yield: *5 cups, 5 servings*

Tartar Sauce

1 cup Diabetic Salad Dressing (see p. 134)
2 Tablespoons pickle relish
1 Tablespoon onions, chopped finely
1/2 teaspoon salad mustard
1 teaspoon parsley, chopped fine
1 Tablespoon lemon juice

Place dressing, pickle relish, onions, mustard, parsley and lemon juice in a small bowl and mix to blend. Refrigerate until served, using 1 Tablespoon per serving.

Nutritive values per serving: *cal 13, cho 2 gm, pro 1 gm, fat 1 gm, Na 3 mg*
Food exchanges per serving: *Up to and including 2 Tablespoons may be considered free. 3 or 4 Tablespoons are 1 vegetable exchange.*
Low-sodium diets: *Use low-sodium Diabetic Salad Dressing (see p. 134)*
Low-cholesterol diets: *Use low-cholesterol Diabetic Salad Dressing.*
Yield: *1 1/4 cups, 20 servings*

Broccoli Fritatta

Dave Christen introduced me to these a couple of years ago and we have been eating them frequently since then. Dave's favorite includes a couple of eggs, 1 slice of cubed bread and 1 ounce each of cheese and ham. I like this version and also a version in which I use mushrooms instead of the cheese and occasionally onions and peppers as the vegetable. You can use a lot of different ingredients as long as you use the basic eggs and count the exchanges for whatever ingredients you add to them.

2 eggs
salt and pepper to taste
1 ounce cubed cheddar or American processed cheese
1/2 cup chopped cooked broccoli

Place eggs in a small bowl, beat them with a fork to blend well and add salt and pepper. Mix lightly and fold cheese and broccoli into the eggs.

Heat an 8-inch frying pan, preferably one with a hard surface, about 1/2 minute over medium heat. Spray pan with pan spray or grease very lightly with margarine or oil. Pour the egg mixture into the frying pan and cook over medium heat until lightly browned on the bottom, turn over and continue to cook, over low heat, until eggs are firm and lightly browned. Serve hot, using 1 fritatta per serving.

Nutritive values per serving: *cal 293, cho 5 gm, pro 22 gm, fat 20 gm, Na variable. This recipe is a good source of fiber.*

Food exchanges per serving: *1 vegetable, 3 medium-fat meat and 1 fat*

Low-sodium diets: *Omit salt. Use low-sodium cheese.*

Low-cholesterol diets: *Omit eggs. Use 1/2 cup liquid egg substitute. Use low-fat cheese.*

Yield: *1 fritatta, 1 serving*

Escalloped Asparagus and Eggs

1 10-ounce package frozen asparagus pieces
1/2 cup egg noodles
1 10 3/4-ounce can condensed cream of chicken soup
3/4 cup water
4 hard-cooked medium sized eggs
2 Tablespoons bread crumbs

Cook asparagus according to directions on the package, drain well and set aside. (You should have about 1 1/2 cups drained asparagus.) Cook egg noodles according to directions on the package. (You should have about 1 1/2 cups drained noodles.) Combine soup and water and mix until smooth. Combine the ingredients in a 1 1/2 quart casserole:

1. 1/3 of the soup mixture;
2. 1/2 of the cooked noodles;
3. 1/2 of the asparagus;
4. 2 sliced eggs;
5. 1/3 of the soup mixture;
6. The rest of the asparagus;
7. The rest of the sliced eggs; and
8. The rest of the soup.

Sprinkle the bread crumbs over the top of the casserole.

Bake at 350°F for about 30 minutes or until hot and bubbly. Serve hot, using 1/4 of the casserole, about 1 cup, per serving.

Nutritive values per serving: *cal 201, cho 17 gm, pro 11 gm, fat 11 gm, Na 559 mg*
Food exchanges per serving: *1 bread and 1 high-fat meat*
Low-sodium diets: *Use low-sodium soup.*
Low-cholesterol diets: *Use only hard-cooked egg whites. This will change the meat exchanges to 1 1/2 low-fat meat.*
Yield: *about 4 1/2 cups, 4 servings*

Macaroni and Cheese

This is such a pretty dish and it tastes so good. It would be a shame not to have it because we are diabetic.

- *1 cup elbow macaroni*
- *1 1/2 cups water at room temperature*
- *3 Tablespoons all-purpose flour*
- *3 Tablespoons instant dry milk*
- *1 1/2 teaspoons salad mustard*
- *1/8 teaspoon white pepper (optional)*
- *3 ounces (1 cup) grated cheddar cheese*
- *3 ounces cubed cheddar cheese*
- *paprika*

Cook elbow macaroni according to directions on the package, drain well and set aside for later use.

While the macaroni is cooking, combine water, flour and dry milk in a small saucepan, mix to make a smooth paste and then cook and stir over medium heat until smooth and thickened to form a sauce. Add mustard, pepper and grated cheese to sauce, return to low heat and cook and stir until cheese is melted. Combine cheese sauce and macaroni and stir to coat the macaroni well with the sauce. Add cubed cheese and place macaroni mixture in a lightly greased 1-quart casserole. Sprinkle lightly with paprika and bake at 325°F for 20 to 30 minutes or until firm and lightly browned. Serve hot, using 1/2 cup per serving.

Nutritive values per serving: *cal 161, cho 10 gm, pro 9 gm, fat 10 gm, Na 198 mg*

Food exchanges per serving: *2/3 bread and 1 high-fat meat*

Low-sodium diets: *Use low-sodium cheese.*

Low-cholesterol diets: *Use low-cholesterol cheese substitute.*

Yield: *3 cups, 6 servings*

Cream Sauces

We used to think that cream sauces had to have a lot of fat in them for a good flavor, but experimenting with different sauces has shown me that isn't really true. A good cream sauce can be made with less fat so that it is much easier to fit into a diabetic diet. Cheese sauce doesn't really need any fat in the basic sauce because there is enough fat in the cheese to give you a good smooth sauce. Seasonings can be varied as desired, using different salts. Onion and garlic salt, celery salt or celery seed, mustard, and dill weed, among others, give a different character to the basic sauces. This sauce is the medium sauce you use for casseroles and creamed dishes. If you want a thin sauce for soups, double the amount of liquid but keep the rest of the ingredients the same.

Ingredients	Béchamel	Velouté	Cheese
Water	2 cups		2 cups
Fat-free chicken broth		2 cups	
Instant dry milk	3 Tablespoons	3 Tablespoons	3 Tablespoons
All-purpose flour	1/4 cup	1/4 cup	1/4 cup
Margarine	1 Tablespoon	1 Tablespoon	
Salt	1/2 teaspoon	variable	variable
Pepper	sprinkle	sprinkle	sprinkle
Grated cheese			1 cup (3 ounces)
Salad mustard			1 teaspoon
Yield	2 cups	2 cups	2 cups

Methods for béchamel and velouté sauces:

1. Bring liquid to a boil. Melt margarine and combine with dry milk, flour, salt and pepper and stir to blend well. Add all at once to boiling liquid and cook and stir over medium heat, using a wire whip, until sauce is smooth and thick and the starchy taste is gone. (A wire whip must be used. This method won't work with a spoon.)
2. Stir dry milk, flour, salt and pepper into liquid and stir to form a smooth paste. Bring to a simmer, add margarine

and then cook and stir over medium heat until smooth and thickened and the starchy taste is gone.

3. Cook and stir margarine and flour over low heat until smooth. Combine dry milk, liquid, salt and pepper and mix until smooth. Add cold liquid to flour mixture and cook and stir over medium heat until sauce is smooth and thick and the starchy taste is gone.

Method for cheese sauce:

Add dry milk, flour, salt and pepper to liquid and stir to form a smooth paste. Cook and stir over medium heat until sauce is smooth and thick and the starchy taste is gone. Remove from heat and add cheese and mustard. Return to heat and stir over low heat until cheese is melted, but do not let the sauce simmer or boil after the cheese is added.

Nutritive values per 1/4 cup serving:
Béchamel sauce: *cal 30, cho 4 gm, pro 1 gm, fat 2 gm, Na (with added salt) 162 mg*
Velouté sauce: *cal 42, cho 4 gm, pro 2 gm, fat 2 gm, Na (without added salt) 533 mg*
Cheese sauce: *cal 82, cho 5 gm, pro 4 gm, fat 5 gm, Na (without added salt) 278 mg*

Food exchanges per 1/4 cup serving:
Béchamel and velouté sauces: *1 vegetable*
Cheese sauce: *1 vegetable and 1 fat*

Low-sodium diets:
Béchamel sauce: *Omit salt. Use salt-free margarine.*
Velouté sauce: *Do not add salt. Use low-sodium broth and salt-free margarine.*
Cheese sauce: *Do not add salt. Use low-sodium cheese.*

Low-cholesterol diets: *Béchamel and velouté sauces may be used as written. Use low-fat cheese for cheese sauce.*

Yield: *2 cups, 8 servings*

Chapter 8

VEGETABLES

Vegetables are very important in a diabetic diet. They are low in carbohydrates and calories but high in texture, appearance and taste appeal. They add fiber, vitamins and minerals and color to our diets. They can be as simple as a carrot stick or as sophisticated as stir-fried vegetables in a sauce.

It is a shame that many people dislike most vegetables and that few restaurants take time to try to make them really appealing to their customers. Mothers do a great job trying to teach their children to eat vegetables but sometimes I think they would be more successful if they would refuse to let their children have vegetables until they had finished their dessert. Who knows, it just might work. Maybe if vegetables cost ration points or were excessively expensive, everyone would value them more than they do now.

We have thought for too long that we were restricted to very plain vegetables with very little seasoning. It is time we learned that vegetables can be exciting. We don't need to restrict ourselves to opening a can of vegetables or throwing a block of frozen vegetables in the microwave oven. They can be steamed, baked, stir-fried or creamed, and they can always be simmered in a very small amount of liquid and garnished with some parsley or chopped chives. In fact, they can add a very great deal to our daily diet.

Frances Nielsen, to whom this book is dedicated, taught me to appreciate vegetables. She really loves the first new peas and potatoes, the first tomatoes and those bright and shining fresh green peppers out in the garden. At first, I was rather amused at her enthusiasm and it wasn't until I had known her for awhile that I discovered in Europe, where she lived until she was eighteen, the new fruits and vegetables are celebrated with festivals and great excitement.

Frances does the most wonderful things with vegetables. She creams them, makes beautiful vegetable platters, steams them, bakes them and puts them in casseroles of every conceivable kind. Since her husband, Denny, died she lives in a suburb of Chicago and has only a very small garden, but she generally comes out to Iowa and spends the month of August and/or September with us so we can enjoy the results of Chuck's garden together.

Some diabetics feel we shouldn't enjoy creamed vegetables but we can if we use a lean cream sauce (see p. 101) and cream vegetables such as broccoli, Brussels sprouts and cabbage, which are low in carbohydrate. Frances's husband always preferred creamed vegetables and we used to enjoy the many combinations that Frances prepared for all of us. I still enjoy them and frequently have a creamed vegetable with hard-cooked liquid egg substitute for lunch.

It is hard to imagine, but I only discovered steamed vegetables a couple of years ago. We had always used a steamer at work, and I thought they were wonderful. In fact, I convinced the auxiliary at the Lutheran nursing home where I worked as a dietary consultant to buy a new steamer for the kitchen. It was a great hit with the dietary staff and the residents told us how much better the vegetables tasted when we steamed them. I have discovered that frozen vegetables need to be steamed about 1 1/2 times as long as the directions indicate for preparation in a microwave oven. For steaming fresh vegetables, the following table might be a guide for you but in the long run, you should steam them until they are crisp-tender or well done according to your own preference.

Vegetable	*Steaming Time*
Asparagus	10 to 20 minutes
Green or wax beans	20 to 30 minutes
Broccoli	12 to 15 minutes
Brussels sprouts	14 to 20 minutes
Cabbage	12 to 18 minutes
Carrots	15 to 20 minutes
Cauliflower	12 to 15 minutes
Onions	15 to 30 minutes
White potatoes	15 to 22 minutes
Summer squash	18 to 25 minutes

I have also discovered that I like to put my steamed vegetables in a serving dish, cover them with a clean napkin or cloth and let them set about 5 minutes. Honestly, they will stay hot and they will lose a lot of steam that way and taste much better. I learned that little trick when I was visiting in Ireland several years ago; that is how they manage to get those lovely dry, mealy potatoes that are such a joy there.

Vegetables should always be thoroughly washed even if you are going to peel them. It is also important to peel them with a sharp knife or potato peeler so that as little skin as possible will be removed. This will help increase your yield and it will also help to keep the nutrients found just under the skin.

Vegetables should be stored in the refrigerator or in a cool dry spot after you get them. If they are kept too long and begin to wilt, you can often restore them by soaking them in cool water, but this won't help restore the vitamin content, which is generally diminished after long storage.

Legumes (dried peas, beans and lentils) are good food bargains. They are inexpensive and are an excellent source of calcium, iron, B vitamins and fiber as well as carbohydrates and protein. They are relatively easy to cook, but please don't try to cook them in a pressure cooker. I did once and the steam vent clogged. The resulting explosion was so loud that even the neighbors heard it, and I'll never forget how ghastly the cupboards and ceiling in our kitchen looked with split pea soup all over them.

My favorite way of cooking dried beans and peas is to cover them with hot water, let them simmer for a few minutes and then set for an hour or so. After that, I drain them well, add more hot water to cover them and simmer them for an hour or so until they are tender. Food exchanges for legumes are listed for cooked weight, so I always figure exchanges on cooked weight rather than raw. Lentils don't need to be presoaked. Just add 5 cups of water per pound of lentils and simmer them for 20 to 30 minutes with a teaspoon of salt until they are tender.

I was never sure of the exact yield of cooked legumes from a cup of dried ones, so I called Patti Dillon, our Fayette County Extension Home Economist. She referred me to their headquarters at Iowa State University at Ames, Iowa (where I graduated) and they sent me the following table.

1 cup dry volume black beans and small lima beans will yield 2 cups cooked volume.

1 cup dry volume blackeye beans, great northern beans, large lima beans, navy beans, pinto beans, whole dried peas, split dried peas or lentils will yield 2 1/2 cups cooked volume.

1 cup dry kidney beans will yield 2 3/4 cups cooked volume.

Another vegetable that is often slighted in menu planning is greens. There are several very good kinds of greens and they are a powerhouse of nutrition as well as a very good source of fiber. They are very low in calories, easy to prepare and delicious. They shouldn't be cooked too long—I like to cook fresh spinach very quickly over moderate heat, using just the liquid that is on the spinach after you have washed it very carefully. I grew up in a German community and I can still remember the long rows of kale in our neighbors' garden. They cooked kale with potatoes and dumplings, in meat or chicken broth, or just simmered it and served it with hard-cooked eggs or vinegar. I still like to serve vinegar with any kind of greens and I still use the little glass vinegar cruet which always sat on the table at home when my mother cooked greens. Mustard and turnip greens need to be cooked a little longer, but they too are delicious and full of iron, calcium and vitamins. My grandmother often talked about picking dandelion greens when she was younger but I don't do it now, even though we have plenty of them, for fear of contamination from some of the fertilizers or weed killers that Chuck uses on the lawn.

So enjoy your vegetables and remember that they can be interesting, and that very few other foods can give you as much satisfaction and food value for as little carbohydrate and calories.

Shredded Carrots

This is more a method than a recipe. It is so good that I couldn't resist including it just in case you don't use it now. You can use the same method for cooking turnips, kohlrabi and rutabagas.

1 pound fresh carrots
salt and pepper to taste
chopped parsley

Clean carrots and shred them coarsely or slice them very thin in your food processor. Place the carrots in the top of a steamer over simmering water and steam, stirring once or twice, for about 10 minutes or until tender. Remove from heat, season to taste and serve hot garnished with parsley. The size of serving may vary a bit depending upon how coarsely the carrots were shredded or how thick the slices are, but the serving should be 1/4 of the final amount of cooked carrots and should be around 1/2 cup.

Nutritive values per serving: *cal 44, cho 9 gm, pro 1 gm, fat negligible, Na variable. This recipe is a good source of fiber.*

Food exchanges per serving: *1/2 bread*

Low-sodium diets: *Do not add salt.*

Low-cholesterol diets: *May be used as written.*

Yield: *about 2 cups, 4 servings*

Creamed Cauliflower

1 10-ounce package frozen cauliflower

3/4 cup cream sauce (see p. 101)

Cook cauliflower according to directions on the package. Cut into bite-sized pieces, add cream sauce and serve hot, using 1/2 cup cauliflower and sauce per serving.

Note: 1 10-ounce package frozen broccoli or greens or 3 cups chopped raw cabbage or diced celery may be substituted for the cauliflower without any change in the food exchange values.

Nutritive values per serving:
with béchamel sauce: *cal 47, cho 6 gm, pro 2 gm, fat 2 gm, Na 139 mg. This recipe is a good source of fiber with any of the sauces.*
with velouté sauce: *cal 49, cho 6 gm, pro 3 gm, fat 2 gm, Na 417 mg*
with cheese sauce: *cal 79, cho 6 gm, pro 4 gm, fat 4 gm, Na 902 mg*

Food exchanges per serving:
with béchamel or velouté sauce: *1 vegetable*
with cheese sauce: *1 vegetable and 1 fat*

Low-sodium diets: *Use low-sodium version of the sauces.*

Low-cholesterol diets: *Use low-cholesterol versions of the sauces.*

Yield: *2 cups, 4 servings*

Saucy Beans and Mushrooms

1 16-ounce can green string beans
1 4-ounce can mushroom slices and pieces
1/4 cup cold water
1 Tablespoon cornstarch
1 Tablespoon soy sauce
1/4 teaspoon salt
sprinkle of pepper
1 1-gram packet Equal sugar substitute
1/4 cup chopped green onions with tops

Place green beans and mushrooms in a saucepan along with their juices, cover and heat over medium heat until boiling. Drain well, reserving 1/2 cup of the juice. Return the juice to the saucepan. Stir water, cornstarch, soy sauce, salt and pepper together until smooth. Add to liquid and cook and stir over medium heat until smooth and thickened. Add green beans and mushrooms to sauce and reheat to serving temperature. Stir green onions into vegetables and serve hot, using 1/2 cup per serving.

Nutritive values per serving: *cal 40, cho 8 gm, pro 2 gm, fat negligible, Na 808 mg. This recipe is a good source of fiber.*
Food exchanges per serving: *1/2 bread*
Low-sodium diets: *Omit salt and soy sauce. Add 1/2 teaspoon chili powder or Italian seasoning.*
Low-cholesterol diets: *May be used as written.*
Yield: *2 cups, 4 servings*

Braised Beets and Celery

My cousin LaVerle Sniffin from Waterloo, Iowa, served this to us when we were there for dinner, and Chuck and I both thought it was the best beet recipe we had ever tasted.

1 Tablespoon vegetable oil
1/4 cup chopped onions
1 1/4 cups chopped celery
1 16-ounce can diced beets
1/2 teaspoon salt
sprinkle of pepper
1 1/2 Tablespoons vinegar
2 1-gram packets Equal sugar substitute

Preheat a heavy frying pan for 1/2 minute over medium heat. Swirl the oil over the bottom of the pan and then add the onions and celery. Cook and stir over medium heat 3 to 5 minutes or until the vegetables are crisp but tender as you like them. Add well-drained beets, salt, pepper and vinegar. Cook and stir to heat to serving temperature. Remove from heat, sprinkle with sugar substitute, mix lightly and serve hot, using 1/2 cup per serving.

Nutritive values per serving: *cal 51, cho 7 gm, pro 1 gm, fat 2 gm, Na 190 mg. This recipe is a good source of fiber.*
Food exchanges per serving: *1 vegetable*
Low-sodium diets: *Omit salt. Use beets cooked without salt.*
Low-cholesterol diets: *May be used as written.*
Yield: *3 cups, 6 servings*

Scalloped Cabbage

1 pound 4 ounces fresh green cabbage
1/2 cup boiling water
1 teaspoon salt
1 Tablespoon melted margarine
3 Tablespoons all purpose flour
2 Tablespoons instant dry milk
1/2 teaspoon salt
1/8 teaspoon white pepper
1 1/2 cups boiling fat-free chicken broth
2 Tablespoons seasoned crumbs

Clean cabbage and chop coarsely. Place cabbage in a saucepan with the boiling water and 1 teaspoon salt. Cover tightly and simmer 9 minutes. Drain well, discarding the liquid.

While the cabbage is cooking, stir margarine, flour, dry milk, 1/2 teaspoon salt and pepper together to blend. Add the flour mixture all at once to the boiling chicken broth and stir, using a wire whip, until thickened and smooth. Stir the cabbage into the sauce, stir lightly to mix well and then pour the mixture into a well greased 1 1/2-quart casserole. Sprinkle crumbs evenly over the cabbage and bake, uncovered, at 325°F for 25 to 30 minutes or until bubbly and lightly browned. Serve hot, using 1/2 cup per serving.

Nutritive values per serving: *cal 66, cho 9 gm, pro 3 gm, fat 2 gm, Na 603 mg. This recipe is a good source of fiber.*

Food exchanges per serving: *1/2 bread*

Low-sodium diets: *Omit salt. Use salt-free margarine and low-sodium broth.*

Low-cholesterol diets: *May be used as written.*

Yield: *3 cups, 6 servings*

Sweet-Sour Cabbage

1-ounce slice bacon
1/2 cup chopped onions
1 quart shredded cabbage
1/2 cup water
1/2 teaspoon Sweet 'n Low brown sugar substitute
1/4 teaspoon salt
Sprinkle of pepper
1 Tablespoon all-purpose flour

Chop bacon and fry until crisp in a heavy frying pan, stirring frequently. Add cabbage to bacon and cook and stir for 1 minute. Add water to cabbage, cover tightly, and steam 10 to 15 minutes or until cabbage is as crisp or soft as you like. Stir brown sugar substitute, salt, pepper and flour together to blend well, sprinkle over cabbage and cook and stir over medium heat until cabbage is well coated with the mixture and the flour has had a chance to thicken the cabbage slightly. Serve hot, using 1/2 cup cabbage per serving.

Nutritive values per serving: *cal 55, cho 5 gm, pro 2 gm, fat 2 gm, Na 123 mg. This recipe is a good source of fiber.*
Food exchanges per serving: *1 vegetable*
Low-sodium diets: *Omit salt. Use 1 Tablespoon oil instead of the bacon.*
Low-cholesterol diets: *Use 1 Tablespoon oil instead of the bacon.*
Yield: *3 cups, 6 servings*

Southern-Style Greens

I have included this recipe, even though it seems easy to prepare and might not need a recipe, because I promised a young southern girl I met in a hospital that I would include a recipe for greens in any future cookbooks I ever did for diabetics. She had been diabetic for several years and thought she couldn't have greens because no one had ever told her that she could have them and that they were very good for her. I felt bad about it and thought to myself that more registered dietitians should pay attention to what their patients actually want to eat when they are planning diabetic diets.

1 pound package frozen mustard or turnip greens
2 cups boiling water
1/2 teaspoon salt
1 1-ounce slice bacon
Sprinkle of pepper

Defrost greens and place them in boiling water in a small saucepan. Add salt, chop the bacon and add it to the greens and simmer, uncovered, over low heat for 30 minutes. Drain the greens well, sprinkle with pepper and cut through them several times before serving them hot, using 1/2 cup greens per serving.

Nutritive values per serving: *cal 71, cho 6 gm, pro 4 gm, fat 4 gm, Na 284 mg. This recipe is a good source of fiber.*
Food exchanges per serving: *1 vegetable and 1 fat*
Low-sodium diets: *Omit salt. (This much bacon is permissible.)*
Low-cholesterol diets: *Omit bacon. Add 4 teaspoons margarine to the drained greens before they are served. (Use 1 teaspoon per serving.)*
Yield: *2 cups, 4 servings*

Sauerkraut with Applesauce

1 14-ounce can sauerkraut
1/2 cup water
1/2 cup unsweetened canned applesauce
1/2 teaspoon Sweet 'n Low brown sugar substitute

Drain sauerkraut well, rinse with cool water, and drain again. Place sauerkraut in a small pan with water and applesauce. Simmer over low heat about 15 minutes or until the sauerkraut is almost dry. Remove from heat, stir the sugar substitute into the sauerkraut and serve hot, using 1/2 cup per serving.

Nutritive values per serving: *cal 32, cho 7 gm, pro 1 gm, fat negligible, Na 171 mg. This recipe is a good source of fiber.*
Food exchanges per serving: *1 vegetable*
Low-sodium diets: *Rinse sauerkraut very well with cool water before it is cooked.*
Low-cholesterol diets: *May be used as written.*
Yield: *2 cups, 4 servings*

Creamed Spinach with Peanuts

1 10-ounce package frozen chopped spinach
1 quart boiling water
1 1/2 cups fat-free chicken broth
2 Tablespoons instant dry milk
3 Tablespoons all-purpose flour
1/4 teaspoon salt
1/8 teaspoon nutmeg
sprinkle of white pepper
2 Tablespoons chopped salted peanuts

Defrost spinach, pull it apart with a fork and place it in a bowl. Cover the spinach with the boiling water and let it set for 5 minutes. Drain very well and set aside.

Combine broth, dry milk, flour, salt, nutmeg and pepper and stir until smooth. Cook and stir over medium heat until smooth and thickened. Add spinach and peanuts to the sauce, mix lightly and serve hot, using 1/2 cup per serving.

Nutritive values per serving: *cal 64, cho 7 gm, pro 4 gm, fat 2 gm, Na 604 mg. This recipe is a good source of fiber.*
Food exchanges per serving: *1 vegetable*
Low-sodium diets: *Omit salt. Use salt-free broth and unsalted peanuts.*
Low-cholesterol diets: *May be used as written.*
Yield: *2 1/2 cups, 5 servings*

Chinese Spinach

1 10-ounce package frozen spinach
1 Tablespoon vegetable oil
1/4 cup chopped onions
2 Tablespoons soy sauce
1 teaspoon sugar
1/2 cup chopped water chestnuts

Cook spinach according to directions on the package. Drain well and set aside.

Preheat a small saucepan over medium heat for 1/2 minute. Swirl oil around the bottom of the pan, add onions and cook and stir until onions are soft but not browned. Add soy sauce and sugar to onions and mix lightly. Add chestnuts and spinach to onion mixture and cook and stir over medium heat to reheat to serving temperature. Serve hot, using 1/2 cup per serving.

Nutritive values per serving: *cal 70, cho 7 gm, pro 3 gm, fat 4 gm, Na 715 mg. This recipe is a good source of fiber.*

Food exchanges per serving: *1 vegetable and 1 fat*

Low-sodium diets: *Omit soy sauce.*

Low-cholesterol diets: *May be used as written.*

Yield: *2 cups, 4 servings*

Creole Summer Squash

1 Tablespoon vegetable oil
1/2 cup chopped onions
1 pound fresh summer squash
1/4 cup boiling water
1 cup fresh or canned tomatoes, drained
1 teaspoon garlic salt
1 teaspoon dried parsley
sprinkle of pepper

Preheat a heavy frying pan for 1/2 minute over medium heat. Swirl the oil around the bottom of the pan, add the onions and cook and stir over medium heat until the onions are soft but not browned. Add squash, washed and sliced but not peeled to the onions along with boiling water. Cover tightly and simmer for 10 minutes. Add tomatoes, garlic salt, parsley and pepper to the squash and simmer another 5 minutes. Serve hot, using 1/2 cup vegetables per serving.

Note: If the vegetable mixture is too liquid, simmer uncovered for the last 5 minutes.

Nutritive values per serving: *cal 42, cho 4 gm, pro 1 gm, fat 2 gm, Na 343 mg. This recipe is a good source of fiber.*
Food exchanges per serving: *1 vegetable*
Low-sodium diets: *Omit salt.*
Low-cholesterol diets: *May be used as written.*
Yield: *3 cups, 6 servings*

Butternut Squash Casserole

This recipe always reminds me of Frances Nielsen and fall. I think it is because she often spends a month with us in the fall when the garden is at its peak and she loves squash and all other vegetables, especially in combinations such as this.

2 pounds butternut squash
2 medium size fresh tomatoes
1 cup coarsely chopped onions
1 teaspoon Italian seasoning
2 Tablespoons margarine
3/4 teaspoon salt

Peel squash, remove the seeds and fiber and cut into slices about 1/2-inch thick. Wash and peel tomatoes and cut into slices about 1/2-inch thick. Layer vegetables in a greased casserole as follows:

1. 1/2 the squash;
2. sliced tomatoes;
3. chopped onions;
4. 1/2 of the margarine dotted over the vegetables, Italian seasoning and salt;
5. the remaining squash; and
6. the remaining margarine and seasonings.

Cover the pan tightly with aluminum foil and bake at 350°F for 1 1/2 hours or until the squash is tender. Remove the foil, stir the vegetables lightly and continue to bake another 1/2 hour or until the squash is lightly browned and almost dry. Mix lightly and serve hot, using 1/2 cup per serving.

Nutritive values per serving: *cal 94, cho 15 gm, pro 2 gm, fat 5 gm, Na 317 mg. This recipe is a good source of fiber.*

Food exchanges per serving: *1 bread and 1 fat*

Low-sodium diets: *Omit salt. Use salt-free margarine.*

Low-cholesterol diets: *May be used as written.*

Yield: *3 cups, 6 servings*

Country-Style Tomatoes

1 16-ounce can tomatoes
1/4 teaspoon onion salt
2 teaspoons margarine
1 Tablespoon all-purpose flour
2 Tablespoons water
sprinkle of pepper
1 1-gram packet Equal sugar substitute

Place tomatoes, onion salt and margarine in a small saucepan and bring to a simmer. Simmer over low heat for about 5 minutes. Stir flour into water until smooth, add to tomatoes along with pepper, and cook and stir over medium heat until thickened and smooth. Continue to cook, stirring constantly, for another minute and then remove from heat. Stir Equal into the tomatoes and serve hot, using about 1/2 cup tomatoes per serving.

Nutritive values per serving: *cal 49, cho 6 gm, pro 1 gm, fat 2 gm, Na 420 mg. This recipe is a good source of fiber.*

Food exchanges per serving: *1 vegetable*

Low-sodium diets: *Omit onion salt. Add 1 teaspoon dehydrated onions and use tomatoes cooked without salt.*

Low-cholesterol diets: *May be used as written.*

Yield: *2 cups, 4 servings*

Stewed Tomatoes

1 slice commercial whole wheat bread
1 teaspoon vegetable oil
1/4 cup chopped onions
1 16-ounce can tomatoes
1/4 teaspoon salt
sprinkle of pepper
1 1-gram packet Equal sugar substitute

Toast bread, cut into cubes and set aside. Preheat a small saucepan over medium heat for 1/2 minute. Swirl the oil over the bottom of the pan, add the onions and cook and stir until the onions are soft but not browned. Add tomatoes, salt and pepper to the onions and reheat to serving temperature. Remove from heat and stir toasted bread cubes and sugar substitute into the tomatoes. Serve hot, using 1/2 cup of tomatoes per serving.

Nutritive values per serving: *cal 58, cho 9 gm, pro 2 gm, fat 2 gm, Na 434 mg. This recipe is a good source of fiber.*
Food exchanges per serving: *1/2 bread*
Low-sodium diets: *Omit salt. Use tomatoes canned without salt.*
Low-cholesterol diets: *May be used as written.*
Yield: *2 cups, 4 servings*

Chapter 9

SALADS

It is a good idea to eat a salad before a meal as you do in many restaurants, because it takes the edge off your appetite without adding a lot of calories—as long as you resist those gooey dressings. It is also a good idea to eat salad *with* your meal, for the contrast in texture and taste. One way to compromise is to eat the salad at one time and a bowl of crunchies the other time. Carrot or celery sticks, cherry tomatoes, dill pickles, julienned fresh green peppers, radishes, marinated mushrooms, green onions and lettuce or cabbage wedges all offer a crisp texture and a different taste to contrast with the rest of your meal without adding many calories or carbohydrates.

I have even noticed recently that more and more hostesses are serving beautiful platters of fresh fruits or vegetables to their guests instead of those gooey little pastry bites which provide at least a hundred calories per bite. I am also pleased to see that many people responsible for professional meetings are serving fruit juices and platters of crunchies with whole grain crackers instead of the ever-present coffee and sweet rolls or cookies. I couldn't count how many times I have walked around with a cup of black coffee in my hand because everything else served was simply out of my territory, and I'm so happy to know that finally we are beginning to be served things at parties and meetings that we can eat.

Tossed salads are a part of this new awareness of healthier foods. They offer a bonus for everyone who wishes to take advantage of their abundant supply of vitamins A and C, their iron and calcium, and their abudance of fiber, along with the lowest calorie count of any type of food. I haven't included recipes for tossed salad because each tossed salad should reflect what was best and freshest in the market or your garden that day. There are many kinds of lettuce—iceberg, bibb, garden and butterhead are among the most common. Romaine, endive, escarole, spinach and watercress can all add more variety to your salads. These greens, as well as cabbage, are all free so you can use as many of them as you like in your tossed salads. If you want to add other items such as a chopped hard-cooked egg, shredded carrots, tomato wedges, croutons, cooked diced bacon, sprouts, various seeds, some chopped fresh mushrooms, a few chopped onions or fresh green peppers, you can count them as necessary. A little of any vegetable added for garnish such as a few green beans, peas or carrots need not be counted. You will know if you have used enough of any one item that it should be counted as part of your exchanges for that meal.

Greens should be clean and crisp when you use them. They should be washed two separate times in cool water. The first time, shake them up and down vigorously and then lift them out of the water. Throw away that water and then do the same thing again. Shake or drain them dry, whichever is appropriate. They should be kept refrigerated until they are used. I like to prepare them a few hours before they are used and then wrap them in a damp cloth in the refrigerator until I'm ready to use them. I keep lettuce, celery, radishes and green onions in Tupperware plastic containers in the refrigerator but I wrap other greens in a damp cloth and keep them in the refrigerator until I need them. Greens can generally be brought back to life by soaking them in cool water if they are wilted, but it is better to use them as fresh as possible to get the largest amount of vitamins from them.

I have not included recipes for chef's salads in this chapter because they are all different. You can use any type of greens you like and you only need to count the other ingredients such as meat, cheese, hard-cooked eggs and tomatoes, olives or other goodies.

However, although greens are free, you do need to count most salad dressings—they can be very high in calories because of the oil they contain. Read the labels carefully when you buy dressings. Just because a dressing is labeled "dietetic," "diabetic" or "lite" doesn't necessarily mean that it is very low in calories. I have some good diabetic dressings in this chapter, but the best thing for a really low-calorie dressing is a mixture of dry seasonings such as some of the salad dressing mixes that are available on the market. Use them without adding any oil to them and you will find they are good without adding many calories. You can also make your own seasoning mix, if you like. Just combine your favorite seasonings such as garlic, onion or celery salt, add some paprika and your favorite herbs such as sweet basil or rosemary, mix well, put it in a shaker and you have your own seasoning mix.

There are some other salads which are free besides tossed salads, such as plain lettuce or one of those wonderful gelatins which are so good and are virtually calorie-free. You can add a fruit exchange to them and have a marvelous salad or dessert which only costs you one fruit exchange. They are so good that I'm tempted to prepare them every day.

I have not included many fruit salads in this chapter because they are so easy to prepare and calculate. We all know how much of any fruit is a fruit exchange and therefore we can combine whatever fruit exchanges we like, refrigerate them until chilled and serve them on a lettuce leaf and know that each person is getting a fruit exchange. One of my favorite fruit salads is one fruit exchange of peaches, pears, plums etc., along with 1/4 cup of cottage cheese, so that I know I have one fruit exchange and 1 lean meat exchange together. You can also add a little chopped onion, chives, radishes, celery or green pepper to cottage cheese and use it for a salad. This combination has been one of my favorites for years and proved to be a favorite of everyone when I have served it for parties.

In other words, when it comes to salads, let your imagination run away with you. Just be sure to use all of the free ingredients you can and count the rest of them.

One type of salad which you have to count carefully is the salad including pasta or starchy vegetables such as beans or potatoes. Bean salads are such a good source of fiber that we should include them in our diet whenever possible, and pasta salads are very good and very interesting, as well as being a good source of complex carbohydrates. Here again we should add them to our diets and use them whenever possible, as long as we count them in our overall diet plan.

Chicken Potato Salad

I like salads which can be used as an entrée for lunch along with some whole wheat crackers and fruit. Turkey, lean ham or beef can be substituted for chicken without changing the food exchange values in this main-dish salad.

1/2 cup Diabetic Salad Dressing (see p. 134)
2 Tablespoons pickle relish
2 chopped fresh green onions or 1/4 cup chopped chives
1/2 teaspoon salt
1/2 cup chopped celery
3 chopped hard cooked medium size eggs
1 cup (6 ounces) diced cooked chicken with skin, fat and gristle removed
1 1/2 cups diced cooked potatoes

Place salad dressing in a bowl, add relish, onions or chives, salt, celery and eggs and mix to blend. Add chicken and potatoes to dressing mixture and mix lightly to coat them with the dressing mixture. Refrigerate at least 2 hours or until served, using 3/4 cup salad per serving.

Nutritive values per serving: *cal 219, cho 18 gm, pro 18 gm, fat 8 gm, Na 462 mg*

Food exchanges per serving: *1 bread and 2 lean meat*

Low-sodium diets: *Omit salt. Use low-sodium version of the salad dressing and chicken cooked without salt.*

Low-cholesterol diets: *Use only the chopped whites of the eggs, discarding the yolks and use the low cholesterol version of the salad dressing.*

Yield: *3 cups salad, 4 servings*

Salmon Luncheon Salad

1 1-pound can red salmon
1/2 cup uncooked shell macaroni
1 cup cooked fresh or frozen peas
2 Tablespoons chopped pimiento
1/2 cup chopped celery
1/2 cup Vinegar and Oil Dressing (see p. 135)
1 large firm head lettuce pulled into bite-sized pieces

Drain salmon, remove skin and bones, break into bite-sized pieces and place in a bowl.

Cook macaroni according to directions on the package, drain well and add to salmon along with peas, pimiento, celery and dressing. Toss lightly.

Divide the lettuce evenly between 6 salad bowls. Mound

the salmon salad mixture on the lettuce using abouut 2/3 cup of the salmon mixture for each bowl. Use 1 salad per serving.

Nutritive values per serving: *cal 190, cho 9 gm, pro 18 gm, fat 9 gm, Na 582 mg. This recipe is a good source of fiber.*
Food exchanges per serving: *1/2 bread, 2 medium-fat meat*
Low-sodium diets: *Use 12 ounces fresh salmon cooked without salt and the low-sodium version of the salad dressing.*
Low-cholesterol diets: *Use low-cholesterol version of the salad dressing.*
Yield: *6 salads, 6 servings*

Tunafish Mold

I like to put this salad into individual molds and use it for salad plates. You can add 2 Tablespoons Miracle Whip salad dressing without changing the food exchanges and it is very good, but isn't clear and sparkling as it is this way.

1 6 1/2-ounce can tunafish in water
1 .3-ounce package sugar-free lemon gelatin
1 3/4 cups boiling water
2 Tablespoons finely chopped green onions or chopped chives
1 Tablespoon finely chopped, well-drained pimiento
2 Tablespoons finely chopped celery

Drain tunafish well, break into bite-sized pieces and refrigerate.

Dissolve gelatin in water, refrigerate until slightly thickened, add tunafish, onions or chives, pimiento and celery and pour into a mold. Refrigerate until firm, using 1/4 of the mold—about 1/2 cup—per serving.

Nutritive values per serving: *cal 68, cho negligible, pro 14 gm, fat negligible, Na 19 mg*
Food exchanges per serving: *2 lean meat*
Low-sodium diets: *May be used as written.*
Low-cholesterol diets: *May be used as written.*
Yield: *1 mold, 4 servings*

Lemon-Applesauce Salad

This very pretty salad is particularly good served with fish because the sweet-sour taste brings out the flavor of fish. It is also good with other entrées.

1 cup canned unsweetened applesauce
1 Tablespoon Miracle Whip salad dressing
2 Tablespoons lemon juice
1 .3-ounce package sugar-free lemon gelatin
1 1/4 cups boiling water
1 Tablespoon chopped canned pimientos

Combine applesauce, salad dressing and lemon juice, mix well and refrigerate until needed. Dissolve gelatin in water and cool to room temperature. Add applesauce mixture and pimientos to cooled gelatin and refrigerate until firm. Serve 1/4 of the gelatin, about 1/2 cup, per serving.

Nutritive values per serving: *cal 48, cho 8 gm, pro negligible, fat 2 gm, Na 23 mg*
Food exchanges per serving: *1/2 fruit*
Low-sodium diets: *May be used as written.*
Low-cholesterol diets: *May be used as written.*
Yield: *about 2 cups, 4 servings*

Pineapple, Apple and Celery Salad

1 medium-sized crisp apple
1/3 cup Diabetic Salad Dressing (see p. 134)
1 cup sugar-free pineapple cubes, well drained
1/2 cup diced celery

Wash apples, core and cut into bite-sized pieces, stirring pieces into salad dressing as they are cut. Add pineapple and celery, mix lightly and serve chilled, using 1/2 cup salad per serving.

Nutritive values per serving: *cal 63, cho 13 gm, pro 1 gm, fat 1 gm, Na 67 mg. This recipe is a good source of fiber.*
Food exchanges per serving: *1 fruit*
Low-sodium diets: *May be used as written.*
Low-cholesterol diets: *May be used as written.*
Yield: *2 cups, 4 servings*

Spiced Peach Salad

1 16-ounce can sugar-free sliced peaches
1 cup water
1/4 teaspoon ground cloves
1/2 teaspoon cinnamon
1 .3-ounce package sugar-free lemon gelatin
cold water as necessary

Drain peaches well. Add 1 cup water, cloves and cinnamon to the juice, bring to a boil and simmer for 5 minutes. Remove from heat and dissolve gelatin in the juice. Add enough cold water to total 2 cups liquid, cool until slightly thickened. Stir peaches into the gelatin and refrigerate until firm. Serve cold, using 1/4 of the salad, about 1/2 cup, per serving.

Nutritive values per serving: *cal 39, cho 7 gm, pro 2 gm, fat negligible, Na 51 mg*

Food exchanges per serving: *1/2 fruit*

Low-sodium diets: *May be used as written.*

Low-cholesterol diets: *May be used as written.*

Yield: *2 1/2 cups, 4 servings*

Broccoli-Cauliflower Salad

Lois Schuchman from Hawkeye, Iowa, sent me this recipe after we had a conversation about good salads. I agree with her that this salad is pretty and very good. You might think you need to cook the vegetables, but they are excellent this way, crisp and crunchy with a good dressing.

1/4 cup Diabetic Salad Dressing (see p. 134)
1/4 cup plain unsweetened yogurt
1/4 cup 2% milk
12 1-gram packets Equal sugar substitute
1 cup chopped celery
1 cup fresh broccoli flowerets
1 cup chopped fresh cauliflower flowerets
1/4 cup chopped fresh green peppers
2 chopped fresh green onions or 1/2 cup chopped onions

Place dressing, yogurt, milk and sugar substitute in a bowl and mix well. Add celery, broccoli, cauliflower, green peppers and onions to the dressing and mix well to coat the vegetables. Refrigerate overnight before serving, using 1/2 cup salad per serving.

Nutritive values per serving: *cal 42, cho 6 gm, pro 2 gm, fat 1 gm, Na 77 mg. This recipe is a good source of fiber.*

Food exchanges per serving: *1 vegetable*

Low-sodium diets: *Use low-sodium dressing.*

Low-cholesterol diets: *Use low-cholesterol dressing.*

Yield: *3 cups, 6 servings*

Barley-Vegetable Salad

3/4 cup quick-pearled barley
1 8-ounce can water chestnuts
1 cup chopped celery
1/4 cup chopped onions
1/4 cup chopped fresh green peppers
1/4 cup chopped pimientos
1/2 cup prepared Weight Watchers Golden Italian Dressing mix or other low-calorie Italian dressing

Cook barley according to directions on the package. Drain well and cool to room temperature.

Drain chestnuts well, slice and place in a mixing bowl along with celery, onions, green peppers, pimientos and salad dressing. Mix lightly and let marinate at room temperature while the barley is cooling. Add barley to vegetable mixture, toss lightly and serve at room temperature, using 1/2 cup salad per serving.

Nutritive values per serving: *cal 93, cho 20 gm, pro 2 gm, fat negligible, Na 285 mg. This recipe is a good source of fiber.*
Food exchanges per serving: *1 bread, 1 vegetable*
Low-sodium diets: *Use low-sodium salad dressing.*
Low-cholesterol diets: *May be used as written.*
Yield: *1 quart, 8 servings*

Coleslaw

What would a picnic be without coleslaw? This is good the first day you make it, but we like it better the second day, so I always make it early if I know that I'm going to want it for some special purpose.

3/4 cup Diabetic Salad Dressing (see p. 134)
1/2 teaspoon celery seed
1/2 teaspoon salt
2 1-gram packets Equal sugar substitute
1 quart (1 pound) shredded or chopped fresh cabbage
1/4 cup chopped fresh green peppers
2 Tablespoons finely chopped onions

Place salad dressing, celery seed, salt and sugar substitute in a bowl and mix with a spoon to blend well. Add cabbage, green peppers and onions to the salad dressing and toss to coat vegetables. Refrigerate until served, using 1/2 cup salad per serving.

Nutritive values per serving: *cal 46, cho 7 gm, pro 2 gm, fat 1 gm, Na 282 mg. This recipe is a good source of fiber.*
Food exchanges per serving: *1 vegetable*
Low-sodium diets: *Omit salt. Use low-sodium salad dressing.*
Low-cholesterol diets: *Use low-cholesterol salad dressing.*
Yield: *3 cups, 6 servings*

Macaroni Slaw

Eva Burrack, Food Service Supervisor at the Lutheran Nursing Home and Gernand Retirement Center in Strawberry Point, Iowa, where I worked as a Dietary Consultant for several years, gave me this recipe. It is good for salad plates and picnics because it combines two very popular salads.

1 cup uncooked elbow macaroni
1/2 cup Diabetic Salad Dressing (see p. 134)
1 Tablespoon lemon juice
2 1-gram packets Equal sugar substitute
1/2 teaspoon dry mustard
1/2 teaspoon salt
1 1/2 cups chopped cabbage
1/2 cup grated carrots
1/4 cup chopped fresh green peppers or pimiento
1/4 cup finely chopped onions

Cook macaroni according to directions on the package, drain well, rinse with cool water, drain again and set aside.

Place salad dressing, lemon juice, sugar substitute, mustard and salt in mixing bowl and mix to blend. Add cabbage, carrots, green peppers or pimiento and onions to salad dressing mixture and mix to blend. Add macaroni and mix lightly. Refrigerate until served, using 1/2 cup per serving.

Nutritive values per serving: *cal 78, cho 15 gm, pro 3 gm, fat negligible, Na 185 mg*
Food exchanges per serving: *1 bread*
Low-sodium diets: *Omit salt. Use low-sodium version of Diabetic Salad Dressing.*
Low-cholesterol diets: *Use low-cholesterol version of Diabetic Salad Dressing.*
Yield: *1 quart, 8 servings*

Sweet Cabbage Salad

This recipe is from Mrs. Gena LeVan, our good friend from Chuck's hometown, Royalton, Illinois. Gena and her mother, Mrs. Bellina, have given me many wonderful recipes over the years. Gena generally has given me salad and dessert recipes, and her mother started Chuck's and my marriage out right with a collection of wonderful Italian recipes, which I'm still using.

1 quart shredded fresh cabbage
1 cup chopped fresh green peppers
1/2 cup chopped fresh sweet red peppers
1 1/2 Tablespoons salt
2 cups water
1/2 cup vinegar
1 cup water
1 teaspoon salt
1 Tablespoon Weight Watcher's sugar substitute
2 cups celery, sliced thin

Place cabbage and fresh peppers in a large bowl. Cover with a mixture of 1 1/2 Tablespoons salt and 2 cups water, mix lightly and let stand at room temperature for about 1 hour. Drain well, rinse with cool water to get rid of most of the salt and drain well again.

Place vinegar, 1 cup water, 1 teaspoon salt and celery seed in a small saucepan. Bring to a boil, remove from heat and add sugar substitute and celery, mix lightly and pour over drained cabbage. Mix lightly and let stand at room temperature for 1 hour. Refrigerate until served using 1/3 cup salad per serving. (This salad stays fresh and good in the refrigerator for several weeks.)

Nutritive values per serving: *cal 9, cho 2 gm, pro and fat negligible. Na about 150 mg. This recipe is a good source of fiber.*

Food exchanges per serving: *1/3 cup may be considered free. 1/2 cup is 1/2 vegetable exchange.*

Low-sodium diets: *Wash salt thoroughly from cabbage mixture and do not add salt to sauce.*

Low-cholesterol diets: *May be used as written.*

Yield: *1 1/2 quarts, 18 servings*

Vegetable Parfait

This recipe always reminds me of Susan Weger, one of the cooks at the Lutheran Nursing Home in Strawberry Point, Iowa, who always prepared it when it was on the menu. When I was working there as a dietary consultant, I was always served the 1,200 calorie diabetic menu for lunch. The food was always good, but there were some things I was especially fond of. This salad was one of them.

1 .3-ounce package sugar-free lemon gelatin
1 1/4 cups boiling water
2 Tablespoons Miracle Whip salad dressing
2 Tablespoons vinegar
1 Tablespoon instant dry milk
1/4 teaspoon salt
1 cup cabbage, chopped fine
1/4 cup celery, chopped fine
1/4 cup onions, chopped fine
2 Tablespoons fresh green peppers, chopped fine

Dissolve gelatin in boiling water and let cool to room temperature. Add salad dressing, vinegar, dry milk and salt to gelatin and refrigerate until syrupy. Beat with a whip at medium speed until thickened, creamy and slightly increased in volume. Stir cabbage, celery, onions and green peppers into the gelatin. Pour into a shallow 1-quart casserole or 1-quart mold and chill until firm. Cut into 6 equal portions and use 1 portion per serving.

Nutritive values per serving: *cal 39, cho 3 gm, pro 1 gm, fat 2 gm, Na 128 mg*
Food exchanges per serving: *1/2 vegetable*
Low-sodium diets: *Omit salt.*
Low-cholesterol diets: *May be used as written.*
Yield: *1 mold, 6 servings*

Chef's French Dressing

I call this chef's dressing because it was given to me by Walter Marion, who was executive chef at Swift and Co.'s headquarters when I was managing their restaurant and cafeteria in Chicago. He was a wonderful chef and, unlike many chefs, perfectly willing, even happy, to give me recipes for any of the good things we served there.

1/3 cup catsup
1/4 cup vinegar
1/2 cup water
1 Tablespoon vegetable oil
2 1-gram packets Equal sugar substitute
1/2 teaspoon onion salt
1/2 teaspoon garlic salt
1 teaspoon paprika
sprinkle of cayenne pepper

Place catsup, vinegar, water, vegetable oil, sugar substitute, salts, paprika and pepper in a jar and shake vigorously to blend well. Refrigerate until served. The dressing is best if it is served at room temperature and should be shaken well before it is served using 2 Tablespoons per serving.

Nutritive values per serving: *cal 23, cho 2 gm, pro negligible, fat 2 gm, Na 247 mg*

Food exchanges per serving: *2 Tablespoons may be considered free. 1/4 cup is 1 vegetable and 1 fat.*

Low-sodium diets: *Omit salts. Use 1/4 teaspoon garlic powder and 1 Tablespoon dehydrated onions.*

Low-cholesterol diets: *May be used as written.*

Yield: *1 1/4 cups, 12 servings*

Diabetic Salad Dressing

2 Tablespoons all-purpose flour
2 Tablespoons sugar
1 teaspoon dry mustard
1/2 teaspoon salt
1 1/2 cups water at room temperature
1/3 cup vinegar
1/2 cup (2 to 3 medium) eggs
4 1-gram packets Equal sugar substitute

Place flour, sugar, mustard and salt in the top of a double boiler and stir to blend well. Add water, vinegar and eggs to the dry mixture and beat with a hand beater until smooth. Place over simmering water and cook and stir until thickened and smooth. Remove from heat and add sugar substitute. Refrigerate until used as desired counting 1 Tablespoon dressing per serving.

Nutritive values per serving: *cal 15, cho 2 gm, pro 1 gm, fat 1 gm, Na 50 mg*

Food exchanges per serving: *Up to 1 1/2 Tablespoons may be considered free. 2 to 3 Tablespoons provide 1 vegetable exchange.*

Low-sodium diets: *Omit salt.*

Low-cholesterol diets: *Omit eggs. Use 1/2 cup liquid egg substitute.*

Yield: *1 1/2 cups, 24 servings*

Vinegar and Oil Dressing

There is hardly enough oil in this dressing to call it an oil dressing but it *tastes* like it has more oil in it, and that is the important thing. This is a basic dressing and you can change the seasonings in it to suit yourself. I like to use 1 teaspoonful of Spike seasoning or one of the packaged seasonings you can buy for dressings with this basic combination of vinegar, oil, water and sugar substitute.

1/2 cup vinegar
1/2 cup water
1 Tablespoon vegetable oil
3 1-gram envelopes Equal sugar substitute
1 teaspoon paprika
1/4 teaspoon garlic salt
1/4 teaspoon onion salt
1/8 teaspoon cayenne pepper

Combine vinegar, water, vegetable oil, sugar substitute, paprika, salts and pepper in a jar and shake until well blended. Refrigerate when not in use but return to room temperature and shake vigorously when used, using 2 Tablespoons per serving.

Nutritive values per serving: *cal 19, cho 1 gm, pro negligible, fat 2 gm, Na 267 mg*
Food exchanges per serving: *Up to 3 Tablespoons may be considered free. 1/4 cup is 1 fat exchange.*
Low-sodium diets: *Omit garlic and onion salts. Use 1/4 teaspoon powdered garlic and 1 Tablespoon dehydrated onions.*
Low-cholesterol diets: *May be used as written.*
Yield: *1 cup, 8 servings*

Chapter 10

YEAST BREADS

Some people think bread isn't good for you and vow to give it up when they start a weight reduction diet. It isn't the bread they should be eliminating, but the butter, jam, jelly and other calorific spreads which give bread its bad reputation. A good honest slice of bread, especially whole grain bread, can be an excellent source of complex carbohydrates, protein, calcium, iron and the B vitamins thiamin, riboflavin and niacin as well as that very important essential dietary fiber. Bread can and should be a part of a diabetic's diet because of the essential nutrients it provides.

You can buy excellent whole grain breads, and they are good for you, but I'm a strong advocate of making your own bread whenever possible. A slice of homemade bread can turn a sandwich or a routine meal into a special occasion, and it disappears like magic at potluck dinners. Homemade bread has more body than most commercial breads—when you bite into a slice of homemade bread, you know you are approaching one of life's most basic foods. I like to cut homemade bread very thin so I can have a sandwich from two thin slices of bread, which only costs me one bread exchange. You can buy thin sliced commercial bread, but it generally doesn't have the body you get in homemade breads.

I love to bake bread. It does something for me . . . gives me some sort of satisfaction that I can't quite explain. I love the smell of freshly baked bread, the sight of fresh loaves on a kitchen counter, and the knowledge that I have created something. I have to stop myself from baking bread too often because we just don't use that much, but I always volunteer to make bread for church dinners or bake sales whenever possible. I'm always surprised that bread sells so fast at bake sales when it is so easy to make fresh bread.

Making good bread is easier than it used to be because now we can buy bread flour, which used to be reserved for bakeries. Bread flour needs special recipes because it absorbs more liquid than all-purpose flour, but it is a help to have bread flour when you want to make whole grain breads. Bread flour is high in gluten, which is low in whole grain flours, so you can get a bread with a much higher percentage of whole grain flour when you use the bread flour. You can't substitute bread flour for all-purpose flour in your own recipes on an equal basis. If you want to adapt one of your own recipes to use bread flour, you will probably have to work with the recipe to see how much liquid you will need to add to the recipe when you are using bread flour.

The new fast-rising yeast is also helpful because it helps bread rise more quickly and can be substituted for the regular active dry yeast with no changes in the recipe or the temperature of the liquid used to activate the yeast (both of them need liquid at 110 to 115°F).

Instant dry milk, which I like to use in many recipes, is also a help in baking bread because you can store it at room temperature until it is reconstituted; it doesn't have to be scalded like fresh milk; it can be added with the flour; and it is generally less expensive than fresh milk . . . and it does add calcium to the bread.

Graham flour is used in several recipes in this book because, although it has the same nutritional value as whole wheat flour with the same amount of dietary fiber, it is ground more finely than whole wheat flour and therefore it gives you a smoother product without that grainy taste which you sometimes get from whole wheat flour. Graham flour can be substituted on an equal basis for all-purpose flour. It only takes 7/8 cup of whole wheat flour to substitute for 1 cup all-purpose flour.

And last, but certainly not least, remember that temperature is very important when you are making bread. The liquid in which you activate dry yeast should be 110 to 115°F. A higher or lower temperature will not yield a good bread and a temperature over 140°F will kill the yeast so the bread won't rise at all. Always remember that yeast is a living organism and reacts like other living things to a change in temperature . . . it slows down when it is cool and dies if it gets too hot.

Sugar provides food for yeast, improves the color of the crust and adds flavor and tenderness to the bread, so we try to use a small amount of it whenever possible. Salt also improves the flavor of the bread and improves its texture by strengthening the gluten. However, if you are on a low-sodium diet, you can make a perfectly acceptable bread without salt.

Cleanliness is very important when you are making bread. Bread pans should be washed well with hot water and soap and then scalded to kill any bacteria which might be present. I use loaf pans with nonstick linings so the bread will come out of the pan more easily, and I like to let the bread rise in a large stainless steel bowl, covered with a clean dry towel. However, any large clean pottery, earthenware or glass bowl will also be satisfactory . . . and they are easy to clean as well.

Knead your bread well. It takes quite a bit of mixing and kneading, and I like to let the dough hook on my mixer work for me, but you can get a good resilient dough mixing by hand, if you prefer to do it that way.

I have used mostly whole grain recipes in this chapter because I am convinced that dietary fiber is very important to diabetics and their families and I want to emphasize that fact . . . so, "Try it, you'll like it."

Egg Bread

This bread dough also makes very good rolls. The dough used for 1 loaf of bread should be made into 14 rolls to yield the same exchange for 1 roll as for 1 slice of bread.

1 cup 100% Bran, Fiber One, Bran Buds or All-Bran
1 1/4 cups water
1 cup water at 110 to 115°F
2 Tablespoons sugar
2 packages (1 1/2 Tablespoons) quick-rise yeast
3 cups bread flour
1 cup (5 to 6 medium) eggs at room temperature
1/2 cup (1 stick) softened margarine
1 Tablespoon salt
3 cups graham flour
1/4 cup all-purpose flour

Combine bran and 1 1/4 cups water. Mix lightly and set aside for 30 to 45 minutes. (The timing is very important.) Combine 1 cup water at 110 to 115°F in mixer bowl with sugar and yeast. Mix lightly and let set at room temperature for 5 minutes. Add the bran mixture along with bread flour to the yeast mixture and mix at medium speed, using a dough hook, for 4 minutes. Add eggs, margarine, salt and graham flour to the dough and mix another 4 minutes. Sprinkle 1/4 cup all-purpose flour on a working surface. Place the dough on it and knead a few times, using as much of the flour as necessary, to form a smooth resilient dough. Form the dough into a ball, place the ball in a well greased bowl, cover the tops and sides of the ball with a light dusting of flour, cover with a clean cloth and let rise at room temperature until doubled in volume.

Turn the dough out onto a lightly floured working surface, knead lightly and return to the bowl, dust the top of the bread lightly with flour, cover with a cloth and let rise until doubled in volume again.

Turn the dough out onto a lightly floured working surface, knead lightly and then divide the dough into 3 equal portions. Round each portion into a ball. Place the balls on a lightly floured surface, cover with a cloth and let stand at room temperature for 10 minutes. Form each ball into a loaf and place in a well greased 9″ × 5″ × 3″ loaf pan, cover with a cloth and let rise until doubled in volume. Bake at 375°F for about 45 minutes or until the bread is browned and sounds hollow when you thump it with your fingers. Turn bread out onto a wire rack, brush with melted margarine and cool to room temperature. Cut each loaf into 14 slices and use 1 slice per serving.

Nutritive values per serving: *cal 103, cho 14 gm, pro 3 gm, fat 3 gm, Na 199 mg. This recipe is a good source of fiber.*

Food exchanges per serving: *1 bread*

Low-sodium diets: *Omit salt. Use salt-free margarine.*

Low-cholesterol diets: *Omit eggs. Use 1 cup liquid egg substitute.*

Yield: *3 loaves, 42 servings*

Light Bran Bread

If you know you need more fiber in your bread but you don't want a dark bread, this bread is for you. The fiber comes from the oat bran and is not all that noticeable in the bread. You will just think that it is a good light bread.

1 cup oat bran
1 1/2 cups water at room temperature
1 cup water at 110 to 115°F
1 package (2 1/4 teaspoons) quick-rise dry yeast
2 cups bread flour
1 egg
2 teaspoons salt
1/4 cup (1/2 stick) softened margarine
2 1/2 cups bread flour
1/4 cup all-purpose flour

Combine oat bran and 1 1/2 cups water. Mix lightly and let set at room temperature for 30 to 45 minutes. (This timing is very important.) Place 1 cup water at 110 to 115°F in mixer bowl. Add yeast, mix lightly and let stand until it begins to bubble. Add 2 cups bread flour and the oat bran mixture to the yeast mixture. Mix at medium speed, using a dough hook, for 4 minutes. Add the egg, salt, margarine and remaining 2 1/2 cups bread flour to the batter and mix at medium speed for another 4 minutes. (This timing is also important because you need to develop the gluten in the bread flour.) Spread the 1/4 cup all-purpose flour out on a working surface. Place the dough on the flour and knead lightly, using as much of the flour as necessary for a smooth, resilient dough. Form the dough into a ball, place the ball in a well greased bowl, cover the top and sides of the ball with a light dusting of flour, cover with a clean cloth and let rise at room temperature until doubled in volume.

Turn the dough out onto a lightly floured working surface, knead lightly and return to the greased bowl. Dust the top of the ball lightly with flour, cover with a clean cloth and let rise at room temperature until doubled in volume.

Turn the dough out onto a lightly floured working surface. Knead lightly and then divide the dough into 2 equal portions. Round each portion into a ball. Place the balls on a lightly floured surface, cover with a clean cloth and let stand at room temperature for 10 minutes. Form each ball into a loaf, place in a well greased 9″ × 5″ × 3″ loaf pan, cover with a clean cloth and let rise until doubled in volume. Bake at 375°F for about 45 minutes or until lightly browned and the bread sounds hollow. Turn bread out onto a wire rack, brush with melted margarine and cool to room temperature. Cut each loaf into 18 equal slices and serve 1 slice per serving.

Nutritive values per serving: *cal 88, cho 16 gm, pro 3 gm, fat 2 gm, Na 136 mg. This recipe is a good source of fiber.*

Food exchanges per serving: *1 bread*

Low-sodium diets: *Omit salt. Use unsalted margarine.*

Low-cholesterol diets: *Omit egg. Use 1/4 cup liquid egg substitute.*

Yield: *2 loaves, 36 servings*

Graham Bread

Graham flour is the same as whole wheat flour except that it is more finely ground. I prefer to use it for bread because it doesn't have that gritty feeling you get occasionally with whole wheat flour and it provides the same amount of fiber and other nutrients that you get from whole wheat flour.

3 cups hot water
1/2 cup instant dry milk
1/4 cup packed brown sugar
1 package (2 1/4 teaspoons) quick-rise yeast
3 cups bread flour
1/4 cup (1/2 stick) softened margarine
2 teaspoons salt
3 cups graham flour
1/4 cup all-purpose flour

Place water, dry milk and brown sugar in mixer bowl. Mix lightly and cool to 110 to 115°F. Add yeast to the liquid, mix lightly and let stand 5 minutes. Add bread flour to the liquid and mix, using a dough hook, at medium speed for 4 minutes. Add margarine, salt and graham flour to the batter and mix another 4 minutes at medium speed. Sprinkle the all-purpose flour on a working surface. Turn the dough out onto the working surface and knead lightly, using as much of the flour as necessary to make a smooth resilient dough. Shape the dough into a ball. Place the ball in a well-greased bowl, turning the dough over to coat the top of the ball with grease. Cover with a cloth and let stand at room temperature until doubled in volume.

Turn dough out onto a lightly floured working surface and knead lightly. Shape into a ball and return to the greased bowl, turning the ball over to grease the top. Cover with a cloth and let rise again until doubled in volume.

Turn dough out onto a lightly floured working surface, knead lightly and divide into 2 equal portions. Form each portion into a ball and let rest on a lightly floured working surface for 10 minutes, covered with a cloth.

Form each ball into a loaf and place in a well greased 9″ × 5″ × 3″ loaf pan. Cover with a cloth and let rise until doubled in volume. Bake at 375°F for about 45 minutes or until browned and it sounds hollow when thumped with your fingers. Turn bread out onto a wire rack and cool to room temperature. Slice each loaf into 18 equal slices about 1/2-inch thick, and serve 1 slice per serving.

Nutritive values per serving: *cal 99, cho 16 gm, pro 3 gm, fat 2 gm, Na 140 mg. This recipe is a good source of fiber.*

Food exchanges per serving: *1 bread*

Low-sodium diets: *Omit salt. Use salt-free margarine.*

Low-cholesterol diets: *May be used as written.*

Yield: *2 loaves, 36 servings.*

Raisin Bran Bread

This is a favorite of my sister Shirley, so I always plan to make it when I know she is coming to see us. It makes excellent toast and is also very good in bread pudding. You can omit the sugar substitute, if you like, but she likes it sweet, so I use the sugar substitute when she is here.

1/4 cup instant dry milk
1/4 cup sugar
2 cups hot water
2 packages (1 1/2 Tablespoons) quick-rise yeast
Sugar substitute equal to 1/2 cup sugar
2 cups bread flour
1/2 cup 100% Bran, Fiber One, All-Bran or Bran Buds
1/4 cup (1/2 stick) softened margarine
2 teaspoons salt
2 cups graham flour
1/2 cup all-purpose flour
3/4 cup raisins

Place the dry milk, sugar and hot water in a mixer bowl. Mix lightly and cool to 110 to 115°F. Add the yeast to the liquid, mix lightly and let stand 5 minutes. Add sugar substitute and bread flour to the liquid and beat at medium speed, using a dough hook, for 4 minutes. Add bran, margarine, salt and graham flour to the batter and mix at medium speed for 4 minutes. Spread the all-purpose flour on a working surface, turn the dough out onto the surface and knead lightly, using as much of the flour as necessary to form a soft resilient dough. Shape the dough into a ball. Place the dough in a well greased bowl, turning the dough over to coat the top of the ball with the grease. Cover with a cloth and let stand at room temperature until doubled in volume.

Turn the dough out onto a lightly floured working surface and knead the raisins into the dough. Shape into a ball and return to the greased bowl, turning the ball over to grease the top again. Cover with a cloth and let rise until doubled in volume.

Turn dough out onto a lightly floured working surface, knead lightly and divide into 2 equal portions. Form each portion into a ball and let rest, on the lightly floured surface, for 10 minutes, covered with a cloth.

Form each ball into a loaf and place in a well greased 9″ × 5″ × 3″ loaf pan. Cover with a cloth and let rise until doubled in volume. Bake at 375°F for 45 minutes or until loaf is well browned and sounds hollow when thumped with your fingers. Turn bread out onto a wire rack and cool to room temperature. Slice each loaf into 18 equal slices, about 1/2 inch wide, and serve 1 slice per serving.

Nutritive values per serving: *cal 99, cho 16 gm, pro 2 gm, fat 2 gm, Na 144 mg. This recipe is a good source of fiber.*
Food exchanges per serving: *1 bread*
Low-sodium diets: *Omit salt. Use salt-free margarine.*
Low-cholesterol diets: *May be used as written.*
Yield: *2 loaves, 36 servings*

Rye Bread

I like to slice this bread very thin so that 2 slices equal 1 bread exchange and then use it with cheese for a sandwich.

3 cups hot water
1/4 cup molasses
2 packages (1 1/2 Tablespoons) quick-rising yeast
4 cups bread flour
1 Tablespoon salt
1/4 cup vegetable oil
3 cups rye flour
3 Tablespoons caraway seed
1/4 cup all-purpose flour

Place water and molasses in a mixer bowl. Cool to 110 to 115°F and then add the yeast. Mix lightly and let stand for 5 minutes. Add the bread flour to the yeast mixture and mix at medium speed, using a dough hook, for 4 minutes. Add the salt, vegetable oil, rye flour and caraway seed and mix at medium speed for another 4 minutes. Sprinkle the 1/4 cup all-purpose flour on a working surface, place the dough on the flour and knead, using as much of the flour as necessary, to form a smooth, resilient dough. Form the dough into a ball and place in a well-greased bowl, turning the ball over to grease the top. Cover with a cloth and let stand at room temperature until doubled in volume.

Turn the dough out onto a lightly floured working surface, knead lightly, form into a ball and return to the greased bowl, turning it over again so that the top has been lightly greased. Let rise until doubled in volume.

Turn the dough out onto a lightly floured working surface, knead lightly and divide into 3 equal portions. Form each portion into a ball, place on a lightly floured working surface, cover with a cloth and let stand for 10 minutes. Form each ball into a loaf and place in a greased 9″ × 5″ × 3″ loaf pan. Cover with a cloth and let rise until doubled in volume. Bake at 350°F for about 45 minutes or until loaf is lightly browned and sounds hollow when thumped lightly. Remove from the pans to a wire rack and cool to room temperature. Cut each loaf into 16 equal slices and use 1 slice per serving.

Nutritive values per serving: *cal 81, cho 14 gm, pro 2 gm, fat 1 gm, Na 135 mg. This recipe is a good source of fiber.*

Food exchanges per serving: *1 bread*

Low-sodium diets: *Omit salt.*

Low-cholesterol diets: *May be used as written.*

Yield: *3 loaves, 48 servings*

Cinnamon Rolls

One day Chuck and I were talking with Vera and Aulden Wilson, and Aulden, whose doctor had put him on a weight reduction diet, said how much he missed having an occasional cinnamon roll. I told him I didn't think either one of us was going to have a cinnamon roll for a long time. However, when I got home I started thinking how much I'd like a cinnamon roll also. So, several days and countless cinnamon rolls later, I came up with this recipe. Each roll takes 2 bread exchanges, so you probably can't have anything except an egg, coffee and orange juice with it for breakfast, but to me it's worth it.

1/4 cup sugar
1/4 cup Sprinkle Sweet sugar substitute (optional)
1 teaspoon cinnamon
1 cup water at 110 to 115°F
1 package (2 1/4 teaspoons) quick-rise yeast
2 cups all-purpose flour
1 teaspoon salt
1/2 cup (2 to 3 medium) eggs
2 Tablespoons vegetable oil
1 teaspoon Weight Watchers dry sugar substitute (optional)
1 1/2 cups graham flour
2 Tablespoons softened margarine

Stir sugar, Sprinkle Sweet sugar substitute and cinnamon together and set aside for later use.

Place water and yeast in mixer bowl, mix lightly and let stand at room temperature for 5 minutes. Add all-purpose flour and mix, using dough hook, at medium speed for 4 minutes. Add salt, eggs, oil, Weight Watchers sugar substitute and graham flour and mix at medium speed until the dough pulls away from the sides of the bowl and forms a ball. Turn the dough out onto a lightly floured working surface and knead several times. Form into a ball and place in a bowl that has been greased with margarine, turning the ball over to grease the top of it. Cover with a clean cloth and let rise at room temperature until doubled in volume. Knead lightly, form into a ball and let rest, covered with a cloth, for 10 minutes.

While the dough is resting, use about 1 1/2 teaspoons of the margarine to grease a 9″ × 13″ cake pan. Sprinkle 2 Tablespoons of the cinnamon sugar mixture evenly over the margarine and set aside for later use.

Roll the dough out on a lightly floured working surface to form a rectangle about 12″ × 9″ and spread the remaining margarine evenly over the dough, leaving about 1/4-inch wide strip around the dough without any margarine on it. Sprinkle the remaining sugar cinnamon mixture evenly over the margarine. Roll into a 12-inch roll like a jelly roll, pinching the long edge of the roll to the dough. Cut into 12 equal rolls about 1-inch wide and place cut side down in the cake pan. Cover with a cloth and let rise at room temperature until doubled in volume. Bake at 375°F for about 30 minutes or until golden brown. Turn rolls out of the pan onto a wire rack and serve warm, if possible, using 1 roll per serving.

Variations

1. Basic Cinnamon Rolls: Substitute 1 1/2 cups all-purpose flour for the 1 1/2 cups graham flour. Food exchanges will remain the same.
2. Chocolate Chip Rolls: Omit cinnamon. Spread 1/2 cup miniature chocolate chips on the sugar mixture when forming the rolls. Cut into 14 rolls instead of 12 rolls and bake as directed. Food exchanges will remain the same.
3. Caramel Rolls: Omit cinnamon. Substitute brown sugar and Brown Sugar Twin for the white sugar and Sugar Twin. Food exchanges will remain the same.

Nutritive values per serving: *cal 197, cho 29 gm, pro 6 gm, fat 6 gm, Na 215 mg. This recipe is a good source of fiber.*

Food exchanges per serving: *2 bread and 1 fat*

Low-sodium diets: *Omit salt. Use salt-free margarine.*

Low-cholesterol diets: *Omit eggs. Use 1/2 cup liquid egg substitute.*

Yield: *12 rolls, 12 servings*

Chapter 11

HOT BREADS

Anyone who is familiar with my books knows that I enjoy muffins and make them frequently, because I always include several muffin recipes in my books. I don't need to make them fresh every morning, because they freeze well and it only takes a minute to reheat them in the microwave oven. Even my husband, Chuck, who worked in a bakery when he was young, and who refuses to eat bread unless it is fresh, agrees that muffins reheated in the microwave oven taste like they were just baked. You miss that wonderful odor of fresh baking in the house, but you can't have convenience and that good odor too, so I generally take the convenience.

When I'm making muffins, I like to use silicone-treated muffin cup liners because you don't have to clean the muffin tins; the muffins come out of the pans easily; you don't lose a lot of the muffin in the pan; and the muffins have a much more attractive appearance when you can get them out of the pan so easily. You can buy them in most good kitchen specialty shops in larger cities. Since we don't live in a city, I buy mine from Maid of Scandinavia, 3244 Raleigh Avenue, Minneapolis, MN 55416. They have a catalog which they will send you upon receipt of one dollar, and if you order, future catalogs are sent to you without cost. I buy the liners five hundred at a time and use them for sticky buns for my husband, cup cakes, individual meat loaves, etc.

At Maid of Scandinavia I also buy ice cream dippers which I use for many things. I particularly like them for muffins. A No. 16 dipper provides 1/4 cup batter, which is used for larger muffins and a No. 20, 3 Tablespoons of batter, which is used for the regular-sized muffins. I have indicated on the muffin recipes which size is appropriate for that recipe. I think that once you use ice cream dippers to standardize your muffins, you'll agree that it's the simplest way to do it.

I first learned to use dippers in institutional work and they worked so well there that I started using them at home. The number on the inside of the dipper tells you the capacity of the dipper; i.e., a No. 16 dipper is 1/4 of a cup because all of the yields are based on that portion of a quart. When we refer to the capacity of a dipper, we mean a level dipper—not the way they use them to dip ice cream, with a lot of ice cream hanging out over the sides of the dipper. Dippers are available in the following sizes:

No. 8	1/2 cup
No. 12	1/3 cup
No. 16	1/4 cup
No. 20	3 Tablespoons
No. 24	about 2 2/3 Tablespoons
No. 30	about 2 Tablespoons
No. 40	1 1/2 Tablespoons
No. 60	1 Tablespoon
No. 100	2 teaspoons

Instant dry milk and instant dry buttermilk are used in these recipes. Baking powder is used with the instant dry milk and soda is used with the dry buttermilk. Please don't try to change them and use the soda with instant dry milk because the soda needs the acid in the dry buttermilk in order to provide the leavening for the hot breads. I think that buttermilk and soda frequently give a better texture than the baking powder and instant dry milk, although there is a special need for each of them in different types of recipes.

Hot breads don't need as much sugar as cakes and cookies, so you probably won't be tempted to add it. If you want any of them to be sweeter than they are, you can always add some sugar substitute without changing the food exchanges.

It is presumed that your oven is preheated and at the right temperature. These are both important for good results and you need to pay close attention so that you will have the right temperature for baking hot breads as well as cakes, cookies, pies, etc.

It is also important to use the size of pan listed in the recipe. You wouldn't believe how much damage you can do to a good recipe if you use a pan which is too large or too small for the batter you want to use. If the pan is too large, the hot bread will be too thin, hard and tough, and if the pan is too small the hot bread will run over the sides of the pan and will not bake completely.

Sometimes different loaves of bread need to be cut into different numbers of slices in order to have each slice equal to one bread exchange. It really isn't all that difficult to cut a different number of slices from loaves of the same size. Read the number of slices required and then look at the loaf. If the number of slices can be divided by 2, mark the center of the loaf, and then you will know how many slices you need to cut from each section. If that number can be divided by 2, you can mark off a further section. When you have established the smallest section possible, make a little mark to indicate the size of the slice and then mark the rest of the loaf to match it. Don't cut the loaf until you want to use the slices, but you will have it marked into the slices you need to cut. I like to use a serrated knife to cut breads of any kind, but I don't cut the slices until I want to use them.

Have fun with the hot breads and remember, if you carry your lunch or are in a hurry for breakfast in the morning, a supply of muffins or slices of a loaf in the freezer can be reheated for a quick breakfast or to carry in your lunch.

Buttermilk Walnut Muffins

I like to keep dry buttermilk on hand because it is much simpler than trying to get rid of the rest of a quart of buttermilk and I don't have to worry about buying buttermilk when I want to use it.

1 cup all-purpose flour
1/4 cup packed brown sugar
1/4 cup dry buttermilk
1/2 teaspoon salt
1/2 teaspoon soda
1/2 teaspoon cinnamon
3/4 cup water at room temperature
1/4 cup vegetable oil
1 egg
1 1/4 cups 100% Bran, Bran Buds, All-Bran or Fiber One
1/4 cup chopped English walnuts

Place flour, brown sugar, dry buttermilk, salt, soda and cinnamon in mixer bowl and mix at low speed for 1/2 minute to blend well. Stir water, oil and egg together to blend well and add to flour mixture. Mix at medium speed only until flour is moistened. Add bran and nuts to batter. Fill muffin tins that have been sprayed with pan spray or lined with paper liners about 1/2 full (level No. 20 dipper) of batter and bake at 400°F for 20 minutes or until muffins are firm and the center springs back when touched. Serve hot, if possible, using 1 muffin per serving.

Note: 3/4 cup buttermilk may be used instead of the dry buttermilk and water, if desired.

Nutritive values per serving: *cal 144, cho 17 gm, pro 4 gm, fat 7 gm, Na 248 mg. This recipe is a good source of fiber.*

Food exchanges per serving: *1 bread and 1 fat*

Low-sodium diets: *Omit salt.*

Low-cholesterol diets: *Omit egg. Use 1/4 cup liquid egg substitute.*

Yield: *12 muffins, 12 servings*

Cranberry Muffins

1 cup fresh cranberries
2 Tablespoons Sprinkle Sweet sugar substitute
2 cups all-purpose flour
2 Tablespoons sugar
1 Tablespoon baking powder
1/2 teaspoon salt
2 medium eggs
1/4 cup vegetable oil
3/4 cup water

Chop cranberries coarsely. Sprinkle the Sprinkle Sweet over the cranberries, toss lightly and set aside. Place flour, sugar, baking powder and salt in mixer bowl and mix at low speed for 1/2 minute to blend well. Combine eggs, vegetable oil and water and blend well with a fork. Add the egg mixture to the flour mixture and mix at medium speed only until the flour is moistened. Add the cranberries and any extra Sprinkle Sweet to the batter and mix lightly. Spoon the batter into muffin tins that have been sprayed with pan spray or lined with paper liners, using 1/4 cup (No. 16 dipper) batter for each muffin. Bake at 400°F for about 20 minutes or until muffins are lightly browned and the center springs back when touched. Serve hot, using 1 muffin per serving.

Variations

1. Blueberry Muffins—Substitute 1 cup whole fresh or frozen blueberries for the cranberries. Do not defrost the berries if they are frozen . . . and do not chop them.
2. Rhubarb Muffins—Substitute 1 cup chopped fresh or frozen rhubarb for the cranberries. Do not defrost the rhubarb if it is frozen.

Nutritive values per serving: *cal 122, cho 15 gm, pro 3 gm, fat 6 gm, Na 136 mg. This recipe is a good source of fiber.*

Food exchanges per serving: *1 bread and 1 fat*

Low-sodium diets: *Omit salt. Use low-sodium baking powder.*

Low-cholesterol diets: *Omit eggs. Use 1/2 cup liquid egg substitute.*

Yield: *12 muffins, 12 servings*

Oat Bran Muffins

Oat bran is high in fiber and good for you, but I had a hard time developing a muffin that we really liked until I discovered that I could use it along with wheat bran for a very acceptable muffin. I think you'll like this one. Chuck says that it tastes like cake but I think it is just a very good muffin.

1 cup all-purpose flour
1/2 cup Bran Buds, All-Bran, 100% Bran or Fiber One
1/2 cup oat bran
1/4 cup packed brown sugar
2 Tablespoons instant dry milk
4 teaspoons baking powder
1 teaspoon cinnamon
1/2 teaspoon salt
1 teaspoon Weight Watchers dry sugar substitute (optional)
1 cup water at room temperature
2 eggs
1/4 cup vegetable oil
1 teaspoon vanilla

Place flour, bran, brown sugar, dry milk, baking powder, cinnamon, salt and sugar substitute in mixer bowl and mix at low speed about 30 seconds to blend well. Mix water, eggs, oil and vanilla together and blend lightly with a fork. Add the liquid to the dry mixture and beat at medium speed only until all of the flour is moistened.

Fill 12 muffin tins that have been sprayed with pan spray or lined with paper cups about 1/2 full (level No. 20 dipper) and bake at 400°F for about 20 minutes or until center is lightly browned and the center springs back when touched. Serve warm, if possible, using 1 muffin per serving.

Nutritive values per serving: *cal 129, cho 17 gm, pro 2 gm, fat 6 gm, Na 214 mg. This recipe is a good source of fiber.*

Food exchanges per serving: *1 bread and 1 fat*

Low-sodium diets: *Omit salt. Use low-sodium baking powder.*

Low-cholesterol diets: *Omit eggs. Use 1/2 cup liquid egg substitute.*

Yield: *12 muffins, 12 servings*

Pecan Bran Muffins

This is a basic bran muffin that I like to make and keep in the freezer. You can substitute an equal amount of another kind of nut or two Tablespoons of raisins for the pecans without changing the food exchanges.

1 1/2 cups 100% Bran, Fiber One, Bran Buds or All-Bran
1 1/4 cups water
1 egg
Sugar substitute equal to 1/4 cup sugar (optional)
3 Tablespoons packed brown sugar
1/4 cup (1/2 stick) margarine
1 cup all-purpose flour
4 teaspoons baking powder
1 teaspoon cinnamon
1/2 teaspoon salt
1/4 cup chopped pecans

Place bran, water, egg and sugar substitute in a small bowl. Mix lightly and let stand at room temperature for 30 to 45 minutes. (This timing is very important.) Cream the brown sugar and margarine together at medium speed until light and fluffy. Scrape down the bowl. Stir the flour, baking powder, cinnamon, salt and pecans together to blend well. Add the flour mixture along with the bran mixture to the creamed mixture and mix at medium speed until all of the flour is moistened. Fill muffin tins that have been sprayed with pan spray or lined with paper cups about 1/2 full (level No. 20 dipper) and bake at 400°F about 20 minutes or until muffin is firm and the center springs back when touched. Serve warm, if possible, using 1 muffin per serving.

Nutritive values per serving: *cal 121, cho 17 gm, pro 3 gm, fat 6 gm, Na 250 mg. This recipe is a good source of fiber.*

Food exchanges per serving: *1 bread and 1 fat*

Low-sodium diets: *Omit salt. Use low-sodium baking powder and salt-free margarine.*

Low-cholesterol diets: *Omit egg. Use 1/4 cup liquid egg substitute.*

Yield: *12 muffins, 12 servings*

Pineapple Bran Muffins

This is my sister Shirley's favorite muffin and I try to keep some on hand when she is here. The pineapple makes it special to her because she is very fond of pineapple.

1 cup all-purpose flour
1 Tablespoon baking powder
1/2 teaspoon baking soda
2 Tablespoons instant dry milk
2 Tablespoons sugar
1/2 teaspoon salt
1/2 cup water
1 egg
1/4 cup vegetable oil
1 cup 100% Bran, Bran Buds, All-Bran or Fiber One
1 cup well drained, crushed pineapple canned without sugar

Place flour, baking powder, baking soda, dry milk, sugar and salt in mixer bowl and mix at low speed for 1/2 minute to blend well. Beat water, egg and oil with a fork to blend and add along with bran and pineapple to flour mixture. Mix at medium speed only until all the flour is moistened. Fill muffin tins that have been sprayed with pan spray or lined with paper cups about 1/2 full (level No. 20 dipper) and bake at 400°F about 20 minutes or until muffins are firm and the center springs back when touched. Serve warm, if possible, using 1 muffin per serving.

Nutritive values per serving: *cal 112, cho 15 gm, pro 3 gm, fat 5 gm, Na 266 mg. This recipe is a good source of fiber.*

Food exchanges per serving: *1 bread and 1 fat*

Low-sodium diets: *Omit salt. Use low-sodium baking powder.*

Low-cholesterol diets: *Omit egg. Use 1/4 cup liquid egg substitute.*

Yield: *12 muffins, 12 servings*

Banana Bran Bread

This bread is so good that you forget that it is also good for you.

1 cup 100% Bran, Bran Buds, All-Bran or Fiber One
2 eggs
1 Tablespoon lemon juice
1/4 cup water
1 teaspoon vanilla
1/4 cup sugar
1/3 cup (2/3 stick) margarine
Bananas equal to 2 fruit exchanges
1 cup all-purpose flour
1 teaspoon soda
1 teaspoon baking powder
1 teaspoon salt
1/3 cup chopped English walnuts

Place bran, eggs, lemon juice, water and vanilla in a small bowl. Mix lightly and let stand at room temperature for 30 to 45 minutes. (This timing is very important.) Cream sugar and margarine together until light and fluffy. Slice the bananas thin and add to the creamed mixture. Mix at medium speed until banana is blended into the mixture. Stir flour, soda, baking powder and salt together to blend well. Add along with the bran mixture and nuts to the creamed mixture and mix at medium speed until blended. Spread evenly in a well-greased 9″ × 5″ × 3″ loaf pan and bake at 350°F for about 40 minutes or until bread is browned and firm in the center and the sides of the bread are pulling away from the sides of the pan. Cool 10 minutes in the pan and then turn out onto a wire rack to cool to room temperature. Cut into 14 equal slices and serve 1 slice per serving.

Nutritive values per serving: *cal 134, cho 17 gm, pro 3 gm, fat 7 gm, Na 180 mg. This recipe is a good source of fiber.*

Food exchanges per serving: *1 bread and 1 fat*

Low-sodium diets: *Omit salt. Use low-sodium baking powder and salt-free margarine.*

Low-cholesterol diets: *Omit eggs. Use 1/2 cup liquid egg substitute.*

Yield: *1 loaf, 14 servings*

Raisin Bran Quick Bread

Chuck tells me that this is his favorite of any of the bran breads that I have developed for my diabetic diet . . . and he certainly has tasted a lot of them over the years.

1 cup all-purpose flour
1 1/4 cups 100% Bran, All Bran, Bran Buds or Fiber One
1/3 cup packed brown sugar
1/3 cup dry buttermilk
1/2 teaspoon salt
1 teaspoon soda
2 medium eggs
1/3 cup vegetable oil
1 cup water
1/4 cup raisins

Place flour, bran, brown sugar, dry buttermilk, salt and soda in mixer bowl and mix at low speed for 1/2 minute to blend well. Combine eggs, oil and water and mix with a fork to blend well. Add the egg mixture and the raisins to the flour mixture and mix at medium speed to blend well. Pour the batter into a 9″ × 5″ × 3″ loaf pan which has been well greased or sprayed with pan spray. Bake at 375°F for 30 to 35 minutes or until bread is browned and the sides draw away from the sides of the pan. Cool 10 minutes in the pan and then turn out onto a rack to finish cooling. Cut into 16 equal slices and serve warm, if possible, using 1 slice per serving.

Note: 1 cup buttermilk may be used instead of the dry buttermilk and water, if desired.

Nutritive values per serving: *cal 125, cho 16 gm, pro 3 gm, fat 6 gm, Na 192 mg. This recipe is a good source of fiber.*

Food exchanges per serving: *1 bread and 1 fat*

Low-sodium diets: *Omit salt.*

Low-cholesterol diets: *Omit eggs. Use 1/2 cup liquid egg substitute. Use low-fat buttermilk, if fresh buttermilk is used.*

Yield: *1 loaf, 16 servings*

Polka Dot Coffee Cake

I call this polka dot coffee cake because the bran in the coffee cake reminds me of polka dots.

- *2 Tablespoons (1/4 stick) margarine*
- *4 Tablespoons packed brown sugar*
- *1 teaspoon cinnamon*
- *1 cup 100% Bran, Bran Buds, All-Bran or Fiber One*
- *1 cup all purpose flour*
- *4 teaspoons baking powder*
- *1/4 teaspoon salt*
- *1/4 cup instant dry milk*
- *2 Tablespoons vegetable oil*
- *2 eggs*
- *1 cup water*

Combine margarine, 2 Tablespoons brown sugar, cinnamon and 1/4 cup bran in a small bowl and mix with a fork or your fingers to form a coarse crumb. Set aside.

Place flour, baking powder, salt, dry milk and 2 Tablespoons brown sugar in mixer bowl. Mix at low speed for 1/2 minute to blend well. Blend vegetable oil, eggs and water together with a fork to blend well. Add the egg mixture with 3/4 cup of bran to the flour mixture and mix at medium speed only until all of the flour is moistened. Spread the batter evenly in a well-greased 9-inch square cake pan. Sprinkle the reserved cinnamon mixture evenly over the top of the batter and bake at 375°F for about 30 minutes or until loaf springs back when touched in the center and the sides draw away from the sides of the pan. Cut 3 × 4 to yield 12 pieces and serve hot, if possible, using 1 piece per serving.

Nutritive values per serving: *cal 121, cho 17 gm, pro 3 gm, fat 5 gm, Na 195 mg. This recipe is a good source of fiber.*

Food exchanges per serving: *1 bread and 1 fat*

Low-sodium diets: *Omit salt. Use salt-free margarine and low-sodium baking powder.*

Low-cholesterol diets: *Omit eggs. Use 1/2 cup liquid egg substitute.*

Yield: *1 coffee cake, 12 servings*

Chapter 12

CAKES

Cake is one of my favorite foods and because of this, I have tried specially hard to develop some good cakes which include fruit, nuts, bran and other ingredients which are good for you and suitable for a diabetic diet.

Fortunately, it is much easier now to develop good diabetic cakes than it was a few years ago. The discovery that diabetics can use some sugar in baking, as long as it is counted, has revolutionized diabetic recipes. Cakes can generally have the sugar cut in half in any recipe without endangering the final product, and from there it is a simple matter to analyze how far you can cut the sugar and fat and still get an acceptable cake. At least one bread and one fat exchange seem to be required for a good piece of cake. The bread exchange is necessary to cover the flour and sugar and the fat exchange to give flavor and tenderness. Most people are willing to give one bread and one fat exchange for a piece of cake but not many people are willing to go much farther than that.

The fat and sugar content in diabetic cakes are cut as much as possible; therefore, it is very important that you follow the recipes exactly. There is little room for error if you want a good cake. You could increase the sugar and fat without hurting the recipes—you might even improve them—but you would be changing the exchange values and making the cake unsuitable for a diabetic diet. If the recipe includes eggs or other ingredients at room temperature, it is important that you take the ingredients out of the refrigerator at least half an hour before you use them. The Gênoise cake (see p. 176) isn't nearly as light if the eggs are cold, as I found out one time when I was in a hurry and decided to use the eggs right out of the refrigerator without allowing them to come to room temperature.

I was particularly glad I had developed some good diabetic cakes when the associate editor of *DITN* (*Diabetes in the News*) called me one day and told me that a young lady had called her and asked for a cake recipe she could use for her wedding. We sent her a recipe for chocolate cake to be frosted with melted semisweet chocolate chips and it pleased me no end to know that because of my testing a bride could enjoy her wedding cake along with her husband and guests. I think that the Gênoise cake (see p. 176) would also have been an excellent cake for a wedding if the bride had wanted a white cake.

In my family you always had a special cake, whatever kind you preferred, for your birthday. My mother even mailed one to me on my birthday the first year I was gone from home to Chicago, and it helped a lot to make me feel loved even if I was a long way from home. I think that I would be very upset if I couldn't have a cake on my birthday, but with the good cakes possible now, my only problem is: shall it be white or chocolate? (Chocolate always wins hands down.)

Most people like to use cake mixes. It is a lot of bother always to have to make our cakes from scratch. Of course we can use angel food cake mix, and I always do, but I haven't really found any diabetic cake mix that I like. One thing I do to make my life simpler is to prepare a mix from my favorite cake recipes and then I can have my cakes in a hurry when I need them.

When you analyze a cake mix or a hot bread mix that you purchase, you will notice that they are mostly flour, sugar, baking powder, instant milk and some preservative. Therefore it is easy to prepare your own mixes which you can keep on hand. When you are ready to use the mix, you simply measure out the amount you need, add the remaining ingredients and have cake in a very short time. For instance you would make a mix for the Black Walnut Cake (see p. 167) as follows:

Ingredient	1 Cake	4 Cakes
Cake flour	1 1/2 cups	6 cups
Graham flour	1/2 cup	2 cups
Baking powder	2 teaspoons	8 teaspoons
Soda	1/2 teaspoon	2 teaspoons
Dry Buttermilk	3 Tablespoons	12 Tablespoons (3/4 cup)
Salt	1/2 teaspoon	2 teaspoons
Sugar	1/3 cup	1 1/3 cups
Dry sugar substitute	equal to 1/3 cup sugar	equal to 1 1/3 cups sugar
Total mix	2 1/2 cups	10 cups

The ingredients must be stirred or sifted together until they are thoroughly blended because you want to be sure to have a mixture which will give the same results every time.

When you were ready to bake a black walnut cake, you would measure out 2 1/2 cups of the dry mix and then add the remaining ingredients as directed by the recipe. This mix should be refrigerated because it contains dry buttermilk, but if you had used the instant dry milk in the mixture it could be stored at room temperature. (Don't ever substitute dry buttermilk for instant dry milk or vice versa. They react differently in the recipe and you would have to change other ingredients also.)

This method can be used for all sorts of mixes. My neighbor Jan Franks makes and keeps on hand mixes for many things—cookies, muffins, biscuits and salad dressing mixes are among the ones she uses, and she is particularly fond of her oatmeal cookie mix. We have often discussed doing a whole book on mixes for diabetics and may eventually get around to it.

Diabetic cakes can be frosted with melted chocolate chips, a sauce, a baked-on topping or a special frosting. Diabetic jelly can be spread between layers and topped with powdered sugar sprinkled on top of the cake (not more than 2 Tablespoons powdered sugar per cake). Two cake layers can be filled with pudding and then sliced. You can use your imagination for other toppings. One of my favorites is the Butter Cream Frosting at the end of this chapter (see p. 178).

You will find a minimum of sugar substitute used in this book because I prefer the taste of the natural ingredients, but if you want cakes sweeter than I do, you can feel free to add more sugar substitute. It won't change the food exchanges established by the basic recipe.

Of course, all the usual notes regarding the preparation of cakes are also important when you are making a diabetic cake.

1. Standard measuring spoons and cups should be used. Pans should be the size and shape stated in the recipes. Cakes can easily burn or be underbaked if the wrong size cake pan is used.
2. Recipes should be read and thoroughly understood before the cake is started. I also like to check to be sure I have all of the ingredients and to measure them, if practical, before I start preparing a recipe.
3. Ingredients should not be deleted or substitutions made unless you are sure they will be made correctly.
4. Flour should not be sifted unless the recipe calls for sifted flour, since there is a different measurement for sifted and unsifted flour.
5. It is presumed in these recipes that the oven is preheated before it is used. Preheating can take from 5 to 15 minutes for different ovens.
6. Cakes may be baked in a pan of a different size than that given in the recipe as long as you remember that the cake pan should be 2/3 full of batter when it is baked. The baking time will also vary according to the size of the baking pan.

Muffin tins are available with a hard surface. I like to line them with silicone-treated liners (see Chapter 11), but if you prefer to grease them, the hard surface is a big help. You will probably want at least a couple of them so you can make muffins and freeze them for later use.

It is also handy to have several different sizes of baking pans to use if you want to increase or decrease recipes. (My friends like the chocolate cake in Chapter 12 so much that I almost always double it if we are having guests.) It is important to remember that each pan will yield a certain number of square inches of cake depending upon the size of the bottom of the pan. Therefore you need to know how many square inches of cake, etc., a pan will yield. The following table lists the more common size pans:

Pan Size	*Yield in Square Inches*
11″ × 15″ jelly roll pan	165
9″ × 13″ cake pan	117
9-inch square cake pan	81
9-inch round layer cake pan	64
8-inch square cake pan	64
8-inch round layer cake pan	49
7″ × 11″ cake pan	77

As you see, a recipe which is correct for an 8-inch square pan can also be used for a 9-inch round pan or it can be doubled and used in a 9″ × 13″ cake pan. If your basic recipe is for a 9-inch square pan you can use 1 1/2 times the recipe for a 9″ × 13″ pan, although you can occasionally double a recipe for a 9″ square cake and use it in a 9″ × 13″ pan if the original cake was rather thin. Of course you must also increase the number of portions in proportion to the number of times you increase the recipe in order to keep your diabetic food exchanges correct, so that if you got 12 servings from the original recipe, and you doubled it, you would need to get 24 servings from the final recipe.

A recipe which fills 12 muffin tins can be baked in an 8- or 9-inch square pan as long as the resulting cake or hot bread is cut into 12 portions to keep the same number of exchanges for each portion. The same recipe can also be baked in a 9″ × 5″ × 3″ loaf pan and then cut into 12 equal slices for the same food exchanges as you would get from each muffin. (You would need to increase the baking time for the loaf.)

Applesauce Cake

This cake is a favorite of our neighbor Johnathan Franks. As he told me once, he is a bottomless pit when it comes to cake, cookies and ice cream. When he first moved next door, I used to give him candy but then I thought, "This is crazy, no dietitian should be giving neighbor children all that candy." So I talked to his mother, Jan, and we decided to stick to healthier cakes, cookies, 2% milk and foods with less fat and sugar in them . . . and he is just as happy with them as he was with the candy.

1 cup 100% Bran, Fiber One, Bran Buds or All-Bran
1 egg
1/4 cup vegetable oil
Liquid sugar substitute equal to 1/2 cup sugar (optional)
2 Tablespoons packed brown sugar
1 cup unsweetened applesauce
2 Tablespoons water
1 cup all-purpose flour
1 teaspoon soda
2 Tablespoons dry buttermilk
1/2 teaspoon salt
1 teaspoon cinnamon
1/4 cup chopped pecans
1/4 cup washed and drained raisins

Place bran, egg, vegetable oil, sugar substitute, brown sugar, applesauce and water in mixer bowl. Mix lightly and let stand for 30 to 45 minutes. (This timing is very important.) Stir flour, soda, dry buttermilk, salt and cinnamon together to blend well. Add flour mixture to bran mixture and mix at medium speed to blend well. Add nuts and raisins. Spread the batter evenly in a well-greased 9″ × 5″ × 3″ loaf pan. Bake at 375°F for about 45 minutes or until a cake tester comes out clean from the center and the sides of the cake pull away from the sides of the pan. Cool in the pan for 10 minutes and then turn out onto a wire rack and cool to room temperature. Cut into 14 equal slices and use 1 slice per serving.

Nutritive values per serving: *cal 124, cho 15 gm, pro 3 gm, fat 6 gm, Na 197 mg. This recipe is a good source of fiber.*
Food exchanges per serving: *1 bread and 1 fat*
Low-sodium diets: *Omit salt.*
Low-cholesterol diets: *Omit egg. Use 1/4 cup liquid egg substitute.*
Yield: *1 9-inch loaf, 14 servings*

Banana Cake

1 cup 100% Bran, Fiber One, Bran Buds or All-Bran
3/4 cup water
1/3 cup vegetable oil
1 egg
1 teaspoon vanilla
banana equal to 1 1/2 fruit exchanges
1 1/4 cups all-purpose flour
1/4 cup packed brown sugar
2 Tablespoons dry buttermilk
1 teaspoon soda
1/2 teaspoon salt

Place bran, water, vegetable oil, egg and vanilla in mixer bowl. Mix at low speed for 1/2 minute and let stand at room temperature for 30 to 45 minutes. (This timing is very important.) Slice banana very thin and add to the bran mixture. Mix at medium speed for 1/2 minute. Combine flour, brown sugar, dry buttermilk, soda and salt and mix well to blend. Add to the bran mixture and mix at medium speed for about 1/2 minute or until well blended. Spread the batter evenly in a well-greased 9-inch square cake pan. Bake at 350°F for 25 minutes or until the center springs back when touched and the sides of the cake pull away from the sides of the pan. Cool to room temperature and then cut 4 × 4 to yield 16 equal pieces. Use 1 piece per serving.

Nutritive values per serving: *cal 120, cho 15 gm, pro 2 gm, fat 5 gm, Na 173 mg. This recipe is a good source of fiber.*

Food exchanges per serving: *1 bread and 1 fat*

Low-sodium diets: *Omit salt.*

Low-cholesterol diets: *Omit egg. Use 1/4 cup liquid egg substitute.*

Yield: *1 9-inch cake, 16 servings*

Black Walnut Cake

We love black walnuts in this area and use a lot of them. If you prefer, you can substitute almonds and almond flavoring or English walnuts and black walnut flavoring.

1 1/2 cups cake flour
1/2 cup graham flour
2 teaspoons baking powder
1/2 teaspoon baking soda
3 Tablespoons dry buttermilk
1/2 teaspoon salt
1/3 cup sugar
Dry sugar substitute equal to 1/3 cup sugar (optional)
3/4 cup water at room temperature
1 egg at room temperature
1/4 cup vegetable oil
1 teaspoon vanilla
1 teaspoon black walnut flavoring
1/2 cup chopped black walnuts

Place flours, baking powder, soda, dry buttermilk, salt, sugar and sugar substitute in mixer bowl and mix at low speed for 1/2 minute to blend well. Combine water, egg, vegetable oil, vanilla and black walnut flavoring and mix well with a fork. Add to the flour mixture along with the walnuts and mix at medium speed about 1 minute or until well blended. Spread evenly in a well-greased 9-inch square cake pan and bake at 375°F for 20 to 30 minutes or until cake is firm in the center and the sides start to pull away from the sides of the pan. Cool to room temperature and cut 4 × 4 to yield 16 equal pieces. Use 1 piece per serving.

Nutritive values per serving: *cal 132, cho 16 gm, pro 3 gm, fat 6 gm, Na 150 mg. This recipe is a good source of fiber.*

Food exchanges per serving: *1 bread and 1 fat*

Low-sodium diets: *Omit salt. Use low-sodium baking powder.*

Low-cholesterol diets: *Omit egg. Use 1/4 cup liquid egg substitute.*

Yield: *1 9-inch cake, 16 servings*

Chocolate Cake

This cake is a chocoholic's dream. It is low in fat and sugar, high in fiber and absolutely luscious.

1 cup 100% Bran, Fiber One, Bran Buds or All-Bran
1 cup water
Dry sugar substitute equal to 1/3 cup sugar (optional)
1 medium egg
1/4 cup vegetable oil

1 teaspoon vanilla
1 teaspoon chocolate flavoring
1 Tablespoon lemon juice
1 cup all-purpose flour
1 teaspoon soda
1/4 cup cocoa
1/4 cup sugar
2 Tablespoons instant dry milk
1/2 teaspoon cinnamon
1/2 teaspoon salt

Place bran, water, sugar substitute, egg, vegetable oil, vanilla, chocolate flavoring and lemon juice in a mixer bowl. Mix lightly and let stand for 30 to 45 minutes. (This timing is very important.) Combine flour, soda, cocoa, sugar, dry milk, cinnamon and salt and stir to blend well. Add flour mixture to the bran mixture and mix at medium speed about 1/2 minute or until well blended. Place in a well-greased 9-inch square cake pan and bake at 350°F for about 20 minutes or until the cake springs back when touched in the center and the sides of the cake pull away from the sides of the pan. Cool to room temperature and cut 3 × 4 to yield 12 squares. Use 1 square per serving.

Note: This batter also makes excellent cupcakes. Spoon batter into 12 muffin tins that have been sprayed with pan spray or lined with paper liners and bake at 375°F for 15 to 20 minutes or until the cake springs back when touched in the center. The food exchanges will be the same for 1 cupcake as for 1 piece of cake.

Nutritive values per serving: *cal 119, cho 16 gm, pro 3 gm, fat 6 gm, Na 224 mg. This recipe is a good source of fiber.*

Food exchanges per serving: *1 bread and 1 fat*

Low-sodium diets: *Omit salt.*

Low-cholesterol diets: *Omit egg. Use 1/4 cup liquid egg substitute.*

Yield: *1 9-inch cake, 12 servings*

Cassata

This cake has always been a favorite of mine because it is so easy to make and keeps beautifully for a couple of days. It is used for festive occasions in Italian families and always reminds me of times in the past when we have served it for special occasions.

1 1/4 cups cake flour
1 teaspoon baking powder
1/4 teaspoon salt
1 cup (5 to 6 medium) eggs
1/4 cup sugar
1/2 teaspoon cream of tartar
1/4 cup water at room temperature
2 teaspoons vanilla
1 pound part skim milk ricotta cheese
2 Tablespoons chopped candied cherries
3 Tablespoons miniature chocolate chips
1 Tablespoon raisins
10 1-gram packets Equal sugar substitute
2 to 3 Tablespoons orange liqueur or orange juice
1 Tablespoon powdered sugar

Stir cake flour, baking powder and salt together to blend well and set aside.

Place eggs in mixer bowl and mix at medium speed until thick and lemon colored. Add sugar and cream of tartar to eggs and beat at high speed, using a whip, for 10 minutes. Combine water and vanilla and add slowly to egg mixture while beating at low speed. Add flour mixture while continuing to beat at low speed. *Do not overmix.* Spread half of the batter evenly in each of two 9-inch layer cake pans that have been greased, lined with wax paper on the bottom, and then the bottom greased again. (Do not grease the sides of the pan or line them with wax paper.) Bake at 375°F for about 15 minutes or until the layers are lightly browned and spring back when touched in the center. Turn the layers out onto a wire rack, remove the wax paper immediately, and cool to room temperature.

Drain any excess liquid from the ricotta, but do not press out any liquid. Discard the liquid and place the cheese in a small bowl. Add the cherries, chocolate chips, raisins, sugar substitute and orange liqueur or orange juice and mix lightly. The mixture should be soft but should hold its shape. Place a cake layer on a plate and spread the cheese mixture evenly on top of the cake layer. Cover with the second layer. Wrap in aluminum foil and refrigerate overnight or up to two or three days, if desired.

Remove the cake from the refrigerator, sprinkle evenly with powdered sugar and cut into 16 equal pieces. Use 1 piece per serving.

Nutritive values per serving: *cal 133, cho 16 gm, pro 6 gm, fat 5 gm, Na 111 mg.*

Food exchanges per serving: *1 bread and 1 medium-fat meat*

Low-sodium diets: *Omit salt. Use low-sodium baking powder.*

Low-cholesterol diets: *This recipe is not suitable. Liquid egg substitute does not work well in this recipe.*

Yield: *1 9-inch cake, 16 servings*

Cherry Cheese Cake

This is a good cake to take along to a potluck luncheon or dinner. It looks pretty, tastes good and provides a dessert you can eat with a clear conscience.

1 3/4 cups (16-ounce can) unsweetened red pitted cherries
1 Tablespoon cornstarch
1/4 teaspoon almond flavoring
12 1-gram packets Equal sugar substitute
3 packets (2 1/2 tablespoons) plain gelatin
2 Tablespoons sugar
1 1/2 cups boiling water
12 1-gram packets Equal sugar substitute
1/3 cup lemon juice
12 2 1/4-inch graham crackers
3 Tablespoons sugar
1/4 cup melted margarine
2 pounds part skim milk ricotta cheese
2 teaspoons vanilla
1/2 teaspoon salt
12 1-gram packets Equal sugar substitute

Drain cherries well, reserving the juice. Add water to the juice, if necessary, to total 1 cup liquid. Set the cherries aside and mix the juice with the cornstarch, stirring until smooth. Cook and stir over moderate heat until mixture is clear and thickened and the starchy taste is gone. Remove from the heat, add almond flavoring, 12 packets of sugar substitute and cherries and refrigerate until needed.

Stir the gelatin and 2 Tablespoons sugar together to blend well, add the boiling water and stir until the gelatin is dissolved. Add 12 packets of sugar substitute and lemon juice and set aside a few minutes until it begins to thicken.

Crush the graham crackers and place in a 9″ × 13″ cake

pan along with 3 Tablespoons sugar and melted margarine. Mix with your fingers to blend well and then pat evenly in the bottom of the pan and set aside until needed.

Drain any excess liquid from the cheese but do not press it to remove any further liquid. Place the cheese in a bowl along with the vanilla, salt and 12 packets of sugar substitute. Mix lightly until smooth. Add the gelatin mixture, which should be syrupy, and mix until smooth. Pour the cheese mixture over the graham cracker crust and refrigerate until thickened. Spread the cherry mixture evenly over the filling. Cut 3 × 6 to yield 18 equal squares. Use 1 square per serving. (Other types of sugar substitute may be used, if desired, using sugar substitute equal to 1/2 cup sugar for each 12 packets of Equal. I have used Equal here because I prefer the taste of it when I can use it.)

Nutritive information per serving: *cal 146, cho 13 gm, pro 7 gm, fat 7 gm, Na 418 mg.*

Food exchanges per serving: *1 skim milk and 1 fat*

Low-sodium diets: *Omit salt.*

Low-cholesterol diets: *May be used as written.*

Yield: *1 9" × 13" inch cake, 16 servings*

Date Bran Cake

Don't underestimate this cake. It is truly delicious, and I'm sure you will like it when you try it. It is good served with ice cream or diabetic whipped topping and it is also very good plain with a cup of tea or a glass of milk. Don't forget, each piece contains as much fiber as most bran muffins.

1 cup 100% Bran, Fiber One, Bran Buds or All-Bran
1 cup water
1 medium egg
3 Tablespoons dark molasses
1/3 cup vegetable oil
1 cup all-purpose flour
3 Tablespoons packed brown sugar
1/2 teaspoon salt
1 teaspoon baking powder
1 teaspoon baking soda
1/3 cup finely chopped dates

Place bran, water, egg, molasses and vegetable oil in a small bowl. Mix lightly and let stand at room temperature for 30 to 45 minutes. (This timing is very important.) Place flour, brown sugar, salt, baking powder, soda and dates in a mixer bowl and mix at low speed for about 1/2 minute to blend well. Add the bran mixture and mix at medium speed to blend well. Do not overmix. Spread evenly in a well-greased 8-inch square cake pan and bake at 375°F for 20 to 25 minutes or until the cake is firm in the center and draws away from the sides of the pan. Cool the cake to room temperature and cut 3 × 4 into 12 equal portions. Use 1 square per serving.

Nutritive values per serving: *cal 138, cho 17 gm, pro 2 gm, fat 7 gm, Na 252 mg. This recipe is a good source of fiber.*
Food exchanges per serving: *1 bread and 1 fat*
Low-sodium diets: *Omit salt. Use low-sodium baking powder.*
Low-cholesterol diets: *Omit egg. Use 1/4 cup liquid egg substitute.*
Yield: *1 8-inch cake, 12 servings*

Dundee Cake

This English cake is traditionally cut in thin slices and served with tea or lemonade. It is available in most stores and bakeries in England, although not in this diabetic version. I like it because it reminds me of having tea in England and also because it is just plain good. I made it once for a lady who moved in next door and she complimented me on my good fruit *bread,* so I'll let you judge whether you think it is a good bread or cake.

1/4 cup (1/2 stick) margarine
1/3 cup sugar
1 cup (5 to 6 medium) eggs at room temperature
1 1/2 cups all-purpose flour
2 teaspoons baking powder
1/2 teaspoon allspice
1/2 teaspoon nutmeg
1/2 teaspoon cinnamon
1/4 cup raisins
1/4 cup chopped pecans
2 Tablespoons chopped candied cherries

Cream margarine and sugar together at medium speed until light and fluffy. Add eggs and beat at medium speed to blend well. Scrape down the bowl. Stir flour, baking powder, allspice, nutmeg and cinnamon together to blend well. Add flour mixture to creamed mixture and beat at medium speed about 1/2 minute or until blended. Add raisins, nuts and cherries to the batter and mix lightly. Spread the batter evenly in a 9″ × 5″ × 3″ loaf pan which has been sprayed with pan spray or well-greased. Bake at 350°F for about 45 minutes or until a cake tester comes out clean from the center of the cake and the cake starts to pull away from the sides of the pan. Cool 10 minutes in the pan and then turn out onto a wire rack to cool to room temperature. Cut into 18 equal slices, about 1/2-inch thick, and use 1 slice per serving.

Nutritive values per serving: *cal 118, cho 15 gm, pro 3 gm, fat 5 gm, Na 86 mg*
Food exchanges per serving: *1 bread and 1 fat*
Low-sodium diets: *Omit salt. Use salt-free margarine and low-sodium baking powder.*
Low-cholesterol diets: *Omit eggs. Use 1 cup liquid egg substitute.*
Yield: *1 9-inch loaf, 18 servings*

Gênoise

This French cake that Frances Nielsen taught me to make doesn't have much fiber in it, but it is a perfect basis for fruit shortcakes which do have fiber. Jan's mother Boots Jorgensen says this is what she thinks of when she wants strawberry shortcake, not the baking-powder biscuits most midwesterners use. Boots's husband Leon is a diabetic; she can serve him shortcake using this cake and strawberries sweetened with Equal sugar substitute.

1/4 cup (1/2 stick) margarine
1 1/4 cups (7 to 8 medium) eggs at room temperature
1/2 cup sugar
1 cup all-purpose flour
1 teaspoon baking powder
1/2 teaspoon salt
dry sugar substitute equal to 1/3 cup sugar (optional)
1 teaspoon almond or lemon flavoring

Melt margarine and set aside to cool to room temperature. Grease a 9″ × 13″ cake pan well with margarine. Cut a piece of 12-inch wide wax paper 15 inches long. Line the pan evenly with the paper, letting it extend up the ends and sides of the pan. Grease the wax paper again with margarine and set aside for later use.

Place the eggs and sugar in a mixing bowl. (It is very important that the eggs be at room temperature.) Beat the egg mixture, using a whip, at high speed for several minutes or until the mixture holds a crease when the beater is withdrawn.

Stir the flour, baking powder, salt and sugar substitute together to blend well while the egg mixture is being beaten. When the egg mixture is stiff, add the flour mixture 1/4 cup at a time and beat at low speed until *partially* blended. Pour the melted margarine slowly into the batter while beating at low speed. Pour the batter into the prepared pan and smooth the top of the batter evenly with a spatula, if necessary. Bake at 350°F 25 to 30 minutes or until cake is lightly browned and springs back when touched in the center. Turn out onto a wire rack and remove the wax paper immediately. Cool to room temperature and cut 3 × 4 to yield 12 squares. Serve 1 square per serving.

Variations

1. Chocolate topped cake—Spread 1/2 cup miniature semisweet chocolate chips over the cake as soon as the wax paper has been removed. When the chocolate chips are melted, spread the melted chocolate evenly over the top of the cake. Score the chocolate 4 × 4 so that it can be cut into 16 equal pieces after the chocolate is hardened. When the cake is cut into 16 servings, each serving will yield 1 bread exchange and 1 fat exchange.
2. Crunch topped cake—Combine 1/2 cup oatmeal, 2 Tablespoons sugar, 1/2 cup chopped nuts, 2 Tablespoons melted margarine, 1 teaspoon cinnamon and dry sugar substitute equal to 1/3 cup sugar (optional). Mix well and spread evenly over the bottom of the cake pan before the batter is added to the pan. Bake as directed in the basic recipe, cutting the finished cake 4 × 4 to yield 16 equal servings. Each serving will yield 1 bread exchange and 1 fat exchange.
3. Chocolate almond cake—Use almond flavoring in the cake. Sprinkle 1/3 cup mini semisweet chocolate chips on the bottom of the cake pan. Sprinkle 1/3 cup sliced almonds evenly over the chocolate chips. Add the batter to the pan and bake as directed in the basic recipe, cutting the finished cake 4 × 4 into 16 equal servings. Each serving will yield 1 bread and 1 1/2 fat exchanges.

Nutritive values per serving: *cal 144, cho 16 gm, pro 4 gm, fat 7 gm, Na 196 mg*

Food exchanges per serving: *1 bread and 1 fat*

Low-sodium diets: *Omit salt. Use salt-free margarine and low-sodium baking powder.*

Low-cholesterol diets: *This recipe is not suitable. Liquid egg substitute does not work for this type of cake.*

Yield: *1 9" × 13" cake, 12 servings*

Butter Cream Frosting

Patsy Spies of Elgin, Iowa developed this recipe so she could make some special treats for her grandmother, who is diabetic. It is good on cake and it is also good on muffins or toast. I think it makes a slice of toast taste like a frosted sweet roll.

1/2 cup water
2 Tablespoons instant dry milk
2 1/2 Tablespoons all-purpose flour
1/2 cup (1 stick) butter or margarine at room temperature
10 1-gram packets Equal sugar substitute
1/2 teaspoon vanilla, almond, lemon or other flavoring

Combine water, dry milk and flour and stir until smooth. Cook, stirring constantly, over medium heat until thick and smooth, or cook in a microwave oven on high for 2 minutes, stirring every 30 seconds. Place container in cold water and stir until cool. Set aside. Cream butter or margarine and Equal sugar substitute together until light and fluffy. Add cooled sauce 1 Tablespoon at a time while beating at medium speed. Add vanilla or other flavoring and beat at high speed until light and fluffy. Refrigerate until used on cool cake, using 1 Tablespoon per portion (3/4 cup for a 12-portion cake; 1 cup for a 16-portion cake). Return to room temperature before using.

Nutritive values per serving: *cal 48, cho 1 gm, pro negligible, fat 5 gm, Na 56 mg*
Food exchanges per serving: *1 fat*
Low-sodium diets: *Use salt-free butter or margarine.*
Low-cholesterol diets: *Use margarine.*
Yield: *1 1/4 cups, 20 servings*

Chocolate Sauce

This semisweet chocolate sauce is good over plain cake or ice cream, and we like it served as a sauce over fresh fruit. You can vary the flavor by adding a teaspoon of rum, almond, orange, coconut or other flavoring along with the vanilla.

1/4 cup cocoa
3 Tablespoons cornstarch
1/2 teaspoon salt
1/2 teaspoon cinnamon
2 cups water
1 Tablespoon vanilla
1 Tablespoon margarine
Sugar substitute equal to 1/2 cup sugar

Place cocoa, cornstarch, salt and cinnamon in a small saucepan. Mix to blend well. Add the water and stir until smooth. Cook and stir over medium heat (I prefer to use a whip for this step) until smooth and thickened; continue to cook 1 minute longer, stirring constantly, over low heat. Remove from heat and add vanilla, margarine and sugar substitute. Cool to room temperature and use 2 Tablespoons per serving. Refrigerate if not used within 2 hours, but return to room temperature before serving. This sauce will keep in the refrigerator for several days but does not freeze well.

Nutritive values per serving: *cal 15, cho 2 gm, pro negligible, fat 1 gm, Na 75 mg*

Food exchanges per serving: *Up to 3 Tablespoons may be used without counting exchanges. 1/4 cup is 1 vegetable exchange.*

Low-sodium diets: *Omit salt. Use salt-free margarine.*

Low-cholesterol diets: *May be used as written.*

Yield: *2 cups, 16 servings*

Chapter 13

COOKIES

Let's face it. Almost everyone we know likes cookies, whether they are diabetic or not, and if they are going to want cookies, we might as well give them cookies low in sugar and saturated fats that can fit into a diabetic diet.

In our area, callers are almost always offered coffee or tea with cookies or cake. This was difficult for me when we first moved out here, but I soon learned to keep a good supply of cookies in the freezer which could be put into the microwave and the callers would never guess they had not been made that day. I try to have cookies that appeal to my husband, who is not diabetic, and to our guests, who are also not diabetic . . . and along with their cookies, I keep a good supply of cookies that are suitable for my diabetic diet. That way I can have a cookie along with our guests without upsetting my daily dietary plan. Most of the cookies are 1/2 or 2/3 bread exchange, and I always save my fruit exchanges for between-meal snacks, so that works out very well.

I think that diabetics should have cookies that have some nutritive value, and I like to include some fiber in them if possible. In other words, I think that if you are going to spend your exchanges on cookies, they should provide you with something more than empty calories. Cookies are a good way to include fiber in your diet whether you include bran, whole wheat flour or nuts and raisins in the cookies . . . as long as they taste good, most people won't question you too closely about their ingredients. In fact, I find that many of my friends are happy to have the lower-calorie cookies as long as they taste good. I've had frequent requests for the recipe used to make my diabetic cookies, particularly the double chocolate cookie in this chapter.

Cookies are not what I would recommend generally for good nutrition, but they can be prepared so they will offer a better source of nutrition than most of the cookies on the market to-day. As for buying "diet cookies," I think they are overpriced and not worth what they cost.

Most cookies are crisp because of a high proportion of sugar, or tender because of a high proportion of fat. Sometimes you have to sacrifice a little texture to get a good diabetic cookie. A diabetic cookie will probably never melt in your mouth or crumble in your hand, but I think you will be very pleasantly surprised to discover what a good cookie you can have using only approved ingredients. It is important not to add more sugar, fat or other ingredients to these cookies, because if you do, you will change the exchange values of the cookies and defeat the purpose of making them. If your family likes a particular cookie and you want to add more sugar or fat, feel free to do so, but don't give those enriched cookies to a diabetic, because the cookies will no longer be suitable for a diabetic diet—unless you have calculated the added ingredients and know how to increase the exchange values for the cookies. You can feel free to increase or decrease the amounts of sugar substitute without changing the exchange values of the cookies. I like a minimum of sugar substitute, but if you like a sweeter cookie, more sugar substitute may be used without harming the cookie.

Of course, when you are preparing the cookies in this chapter, you should follow all of the basic directions for preparing cookies.

1. Read the recipe through and be sure you understand all of it before starting to get your ingredients together.
2. Have all of your ingredients out and measured before you start mixing the ingredients. Have your utensils clean and ready and your cookie sheets sprayed with pan spray or lined with aluminum foil.
3. Do not undermix or overmix the dough.
4. Portion the dough as directed in the recipe. If your cookie is too large or too small, the food exchanges will not be correct for each cookie, because they were calculated using a certain size cookie. I have suggested that you use dippers to portion your cookies. A No. 60 dipper is equal to 1 Tablespoon dough and a No. 40 dipper is equal to 1 1/2 Tablespoons dough. Dippers are discussed in more detail in Chapter 11, Hot Breads. They are a very important help when you are making cookies.
5. Remove the cookies from the hot cookie sheets as soon as you take them out of the oven, because they will continue to cook if left on the hot cookie sheets. I generally line my pans with aluminum foil and then I just slide the foil and the cookies off the pans onto the wire rack to cool until I can handle them.
6. If you don't have a full pan of cookies, place the cookies you do have in the center of the pan so they will bake evenly. All cookies on a cookie sheet should be the same size so they will bake evenly.
7. Follow the recipe exactly the first time you prepare the cookies. If you want to change the method later, feel free to do so, but follow it to the letter when you make them the first time, and remember—don't add ingredients without calculating them in the final exchange values.

Double Chocolate Cookies

These are Johnathan's favorite cookies, which I try to keep on hand in the freezer for him. He even asked his mother to make them for him to take to school for a treat on his birthday last year.

1 cup 100% Bran, Fiber One, Bran Buds or All-Bran
1/3 cup water
1/2 cup (2 to 3 medium) eggs
2 teaspoons vanilla
1 teaspoon chocolate flavoring
1/3 cup vegetable oil
Sugar substitute equal to 3 Tablespoons sugar (optional)
1 cup all-purpose flour
1/4 cup cocoa
2 Tablespoons instant dry milk
1/2 teaspoon soda
1/2 teaspoon baking powder
1/2 teaspoon salt
1/4 cup sugar
1/2 cup miniature chocolate chips

Place bran, water, eggs, vanilla, chocolate flavoring, oil and sugar substitute in a bowl. Mix lightly and let stand at room temperature for 30 to 45 minutes. (This timing is very important.) Place flour, cocoa, dry milk, soda, baking powder, salt and sugar in a mixer bowl and mix at low speed for 1/2 minute to blend well. Add the bran mixture to the flour mixture and beat at medium speed only to blend well. Stir the chips into the mixture and drop by level tablespoonful (No. 60 dipper) onto cookie sheets which have been sprayed with pan spray or lined with aluminum foil. Bake at 350°F for about 10 minutes or until almost firm. (Watch them carefully; they burn easily.) Remove the cookies from the sheet onto wire racks to cool. Use 1 cookie per serving.

Note: If the cookies are made without chocolate chips, each cookie will yield 1/2 bread and 1 fat exchanges.

Nutritive values per serving: *cal 90, cho 10 gm, pro 2 gm, fat 5 gm, Na 59 mg. This recipe is a good source of fiber.*

Food exchanges per serving: *2/3 bread and 1 fat*

Low-sodium diets: *Omit salt. Use low-sodium baking powder.*

Low-cholesterol diets: *Omit eggs. Use 1/2 cup liquid egg substitute.*

Yield: *24 cookies, 24 servings*

Chocolate Oat Bran Cookies with Chocolate Chips

Oat bran cereal has proved to be so valuable in helping to lower blood sugar that I thought we should use it in cookies also.

1/2 cup oat bran cereal
1/2 cup water at room temperature
1/2 cup (1 stick) margarine
1/3 cup sugar
1 Tablespoon Weight Watchers sugar substitute
1/2 cup (3 to 4 medium) egg whites
2 teaspoons vanilla
2 cups all-purpose flour
1/3 cup cocoa
1 teaspoon soda
2 Tablespoons dry buttermilk
1/2 teaspoon salt
2/3 cup miniature chocolate chips

Mix oat bran and water and let stand at room temperature for 30 to 45 minutes. (This timing is very important.) Cream margarine, sugar and sugar substitute together until light and fluffy. Add egg whites and vanilla and mix at medium speed for 1/2 minute. Scrape down the bowl. Stir flour, cocoa, soda, dry buttermilk and salt together to blend well, add to the creamed mixture along with the oat bran mixture and mix at medium speed to blend. Add chocolate chips to dough and drop by Tablespoonful (level No. 60 dipper) onto cookie sheets that have been sprayed with pan spray or lined with aluminum foil. Bake at 375°F for 12 minutes. (The cookies will not be crisp if they are not baked the full length of time.) Remove from hot cookie sheets to wire racks to cool. Use 1 cookie per serving.

Nutritive values per serving: *cal 80, cho 10 gm, pro 2 gm, fat 5 gm, Na 95 mg. This recipe is a good source of fiber.*

Food exchanges per serving: *2/3 bread and 1 fat*

Low-sodium diets: *Omit salt. Use salt-free margarine.*

Low-cholesterol diets: *May be used as written.*

Yield: *36 cookies, 36 servings*

Coconut Chocolate Chip Cookies

These are among my favorite cookies. I like coconut and I'm a chocoholic so I enjoy the combination. They are also a good source of fiber.

1 cup 100% Bran, Fiber One, Bran Buds or All-Bran
1/3 cup water
1/4 cup (2 to 3 medium) egg whites
1/4 cup vegetable oil
1/2 cup sugar
1 teaspoon vanilla
1 teaspoon coconut flavoring
1 cup all-purpose flour
1/2 teaspoon baking powder
1/2 teaspoon baking soda
1/2 teaspoon salt
2 Tablespoons instant dry milk
dry sugar substitute equal to 1/4 cup sugar (optional)
1/2 cup miniature chocolate chips
1/2 cup shredded coconut

Place bran, water, egg whites, vegetable oil, sugar, vanilla and coconut flavoring in a small bowl. Mix well and let stand at room temperature for 30 to 45 minutes. (This timing is very important.) Place flour, baking powder, soda, salt, dry milk and sugar substitute in mixer bowl. Mix at low speed for 1/2 minute to blend well. Add the bran mixture to the flour mixture and mix at medium speed until all of the flour is moistened. Add chocolate chips and coconut to dough and drop by the Tablespoonful (No. 60 dipper) onto cookie sheets that have been sprayed with pan spray or lined with aluminum foil. Press each cookie down lightly with the back of a Tablespoon or your fingers dipped in cold water. Bake at 375°F 10 to 12 minutes or until lightly browned. Remove cookies from hot sheets to wire rack to cool to room temperature. Use 1 cookie per serving.

Nutritive values per serving: *cal 84, cho 10 gm, pro 1 gm, fat 5 gm, Na 106 mg. This recipe is a good source of fiber.*

Food exchanges per serving: *2/3 bread and 1 fat*

Low-sodium diets: *Omit salt. Use low-sodium baking powder.*

Low-cholesterol diets: *This recipe is not suitable because of the coconut.*

Yield: *24 cookies, 24 servings*

Coconut Oatmeal Cookies

Vicki Aylesworth, who grew up next door to us, is in college studying to be a dietitian. When she was in 4-H she used this recipe for a foods project to show how recipes could be modified for use in different diets. She won a blue ribbon with her project at the Iowa State Fair.

3/4 cup (1 1/2 sticks) margarine
1/2 cup packed brown sugar
2 teaspoons Weight Watchers sugar substitute
1/2 cup (4 to 5 medium) egg whites
1 teaspoon vanilla
1 teaspoon coconut flavoring
2 teaspoons lemon juice
2 cups all purpose flour
1 teaspoon baking soda
1 cup Wheaties cereal
1/2 cup rolled oats
1 1/2 cups shredded coconut

Cream margarine, brown sugar and sugar substitute together until light and fluffy. Add egg whites, vanilla, coconut flavoring and lemon juice and mix at medium speed for 1/2 minute. Scrape down the bowl. Stir flour and soda together to blend and add to creamed mixture. Mix at medium speed to blend. Add Wheaties, oatmeal and coconut and mix to blend. Drop by level Tablespoonful (No. 60 dipper) onto cookie sheets that have been sprayed with pan spray or lined with aluminum foil. Dip your fingers in cold water and press the dough down to form a cookie about 2 1/2 inches across. Bake at 375°F for about 10 to 12 minutes or until lightly browned. (It is important that the cookies be lightly browned to develop their best flavor.) Remove cookies from hot cookie sheets to wire rack to cool to room temperature. Use 1 cookie per serving.

Nutritive values per serving: *cal 99, cho 11 gm, pro 2 gm, fat 5 gm, Na 100 mg*
Food exchanges per serving: *2/3 bread and 1 fat*
Low-sodium diets: *Use salt-free margarine.*
Low-cholesterol diets: *This recipe is not suitable because of the coconut.*
Yield: *36 cookies, 36 servings*

Raisin Spice Cookies

Kathy Fassbinder of Elgin, Iowa, took one bite of this cookie and said it reminded her of her grandmother's cookies. We finally decided it was the cardamom in the cookie. Kathy said she hadn't tasted cardamom since she was a child but she was going to get some so her cookies would taste like her grandmother's cookies.

3/4 cup (1 1/2 sticks) margarine
1/3 cup packed brown sugar
2 medium eggs
1 Tablespoon lemon juice
2 teaspoons vanilla
2 cups all-purpose flour
1/2 teaspoon baking soda
1/2 teaspoon baking powder
1/2 teaspoon salt
1 teaspoon cinnamon
1/2 teaspoon cardamom
2 Tablespoons water
1/2 cup raisins

Cream margarine and brown sugar together in mixer bowl until light and fluffy. Add eggs, lemon juice and vanilla and mix at medium speed for 1/2 minute. Scrape down the bowl. Stir flour, soda, baking powder, salt, cinnamon and cardamom together to blend well. Add to creamed mixture along with water and mix at medium speed to blend. Drop by the Tablespoonful (No. 60 dipper) onto cookie sheets sprayed with pan spray or lined with aluminum foil. Push the dough down with the back of a spoon or your fingers dipped in cold water to form a circle about 2 1/2 inches in diameter. Bake at 375°F for 10 to 12 minutes or until lightly browned. Remove hot cookies from cookie sheets to wire rack to cool to room temperature. Use 1 cookie per serving.

Nutritive values per serving: *cal 94, cho 11 gm, pro 1 gm, fat 5 gm, Na 117 mg*

Food exchanges per serving: *1/2 bread and 1 fat*

Low-sodium diets: *Omit salt. Use low-sodium baking powder and salt-free margarine.*

Low-cholesterol diets: *Omit eggs. Use 1/2 cup liquid egg substitute.*

Yield: *24 cookies, 24 servings*

Vera's Oat Bran Cookies

I call these Vera's cookies because they are based on a recipe for oatmeal cookies that Vera Wilson gave me several years ago. Oatmeal cookies were a special favorite of her children when they were growing up, and she still makes them when they come home for a visit.

1/2 cup (1 stick) margarine
1/3 cup brown sugar
1 1/2 teaspoons Sweet 'n Low brown sugar substitute
1/2 cup (2 to 3 medium) eggs
1 teaspoon vanilla
1 cup all-purpose flour

1 cup oat bran cereal
1/2 teaspoon baking powder
1/2 teaspoon baking soda
1/2 teaspoon salt
1 teaspoon cinnamon
1/3 cup raisins
1/4 cup water

Cream margarine and sugar together at medium speed until light and fluffy. Add sugar substitute, eggs and vanilla to creamed mixture and mix at medium speed for 1/2 minute. Scrape down the bowl. Stir flour, oat bran, baking powder, soda, salt and cinnamon together to blend and add to creamed mixture along with raisins and water. Mix at medium speed until blended. Drop by the Tablespoon (No. 60 dipper) onto cookie sheets that have been sprayed with pan spray or lined with aluminum foil. Dip your fingers in cold water and press the dough down to form a round cookie about 2 1/2 inches across. Bake at 375°F for 10 to 12 minutes or until lightly browned on the bottom. Remove cookies from hot cookie sheets to wire racks to cool to room temperature and serve 1 cookie per serving.

Nutritive values per serving: *cal 90, cho 10 gm, pro 2 gm, fat 5 gm, Na 128 mg. This recipe is a good source of fiber.*

Food exchanges per serving: *2/3 bread and 1 fat*

Low-sodium diets: *Omit salt. Use salt-free margarine and low-sodium baking powder.*

Low-cholesterol diets: *Omit eggs. Use 1/2 cup egg whites.*

Yield: *24 cookies, 24 servings*

Chapter 14

PIES AND PUDDINGS

If you have ever doubted that the midwest is pie country you only need to attend one of our many annual church dinners in the fall to realize how many different kinds of pies are available. Cecil Moats and I always cut and serve the pies at our annual church dinner and I find the variety unbelievable. There will be as many as five different kinds of chocolate pie, and you wouldn't believe the variety of apple pies diners can choose from.

My husband Chuck loves pies but I am afraid that I haven't made many of them in the last few years. Pie just didn't fit into a diabetic diet and I had lost my enthusiasm for them, but now that we can have more complex carbohydrate in our diets, pies and puddings have become a reality again. The new puddings and fruit gelatins available made with Equal sugar substitute are so much better than the old ones that I have discovered a whole new world of pie fillings.

Fruit fillings are also good for you, and now, with Equal available, they can be really excellent.

Graham cracker crust has less carbohydrate and fat in it than a regular pie crust, but even a regular pie crust can be a source of fiber, so it isn't all bad. Sometimes I serve the pie fillings as puddings which also reduces their exchange values. I find that I can fit a pie with a graham cracker crust easily into a dinner or luncheon menu and a pie with a regular crust into a menu without too much trouble. Puddings are also a good ending to a meal and can be served frequently.

Graham Cracker Crust

I like to use this crust because it is lower in exchanges, complements so many fillings and is easy to prepare. You can make several and freeze them until needed. In an emergency you can always fill one of them with ice cream or diabetic pudding and have a very good dessert that will appeal to any unexpected guests.

8 crushed graham crackers (2 1/4-inch squares)
1/2 teaspoon Sweet 'n Low brown sugar substitute
1/2 teaspoon cinnamon
2 Tablespoons sugar
3 Tablespoons margarine

Crush graham crackers (I put them in a plastic bag and crush them with my rolling pin), add sugar substitute, cinnamon and sugar and mix to blend well. Melt margarine in a 9-inch pie tin. Add the crumb mixture to the margarine and mix to blend well. Press the crumb mixture evenly over the bottom and sides of the pie tin. Bake at 350°F for 6 minutes and then cool to room temperature.

Nutritive values per serving:
1/6 pie crust: *cal 104, cho 11 gm, pro 1 gm, fat 7 gm, Na 130 mg*
1/8 pie crust: *cal 78, cho 8 gm, pro 1 gm, fat 5 gm, Na 98 mg*

Food exchanges per serving:
1/6 pie crust: *2/3 bread and 1 fat*
1/8 pie crust: *1/2 bread and 1 fat*
Low-sodium diets: *May be used as written.*
Low-cholesterol diets: *May be used as written.*
Yield: *1 9-inch pie crust, 6 or 8 servings*

Oat Bran Pie Crust

This crust is not only good, it is an excellent source of fiber without a strong taste of bran.

3/4 cup all-purpose flour
1/2 cup oat bran cereal
1/2 teaspoon salt
1 Tablespoon brown sugar
1/3 cup (2/3 stick) chilled margarine
3 Tablespoons very cold water

Stir flour, oat bran, salt and brown sugar together to blend well. Cut the margarine into the flour mixture to form a coarse meal. Add water to the mixture and stir with a fork until the dough forms a ball. Knead several times on a lightly floured working surface and round into a ball. Roll crust out on lightly floured surface to form a circle. Fit into 9-inch pie pan and prick the bottom 5 or 6 times with a fork. Bake at 425°F for 12 to 15 minutes or until lightly browned. Cool and fill with cool filling or fill the unbaked crust and bake according to directions for the filling. Serve 1/6 of the crust per serving.

Nutritive values per serving: *cal 179, cho 17 gm, pro 3 gm, fat 11 gm, Na 293 mg. This recipe is a good source of fiber.*
Food exchanges per serving: *1 bread and 2 fat*
Low-sodium diets: *Omit salt. Use salt-free margarine.*
Low-cholesterol diets: *May be used as written.*
Yield: *1 9-inch pie crust, 6 servings*

Basic Fruit Filling

1 16-ounce can unsweetened fruit such as apples, apricots, cherries, fruit cocktail, peaches, pears or pineapple
1 cup liquid drained from the fruit
1 1/2 Tablespoons cornstarch
1/4 teaspoon almond flavoring
dry sugar substitute equal to 1/2 cup sugar
diabetic whipped topping (optional)

Drain fruit well, reserving 1 cup liquid. Set fruit aside for later use at room temperature. Combine liquid and cornstarch and stir until smooth. Cook and stir liquid over medium heat until thickened and clear. Remove from heat and add flavoring and sugar substitute, mix well and then fold the fruit into the cooked mixture. Spread evenly in a prebaked pie crust and chill until firm. Cut into 6 or 8 equal pieces and use 1 piece per serving. Garnish with whipped topping, if desired.

Nutritive values per serving:
1/6 pie: *cal 44, cho 10 gm, pro 1 gm, fat negligible, Na 5 mg*
1/8 pie: *cal 33, cho 8 gm, pro 1 gm, fat negligible, Na 4 mg*

Food exchanges per serving:
1/6 pie: *2/3 bread*
1/8 pie: *1/2 bread*
Low-sodium diets: *May be used as written.*
Low-cholesterol diets: *May be used as written.*
Yield: *filling for 1 9-inch pie, 6 or 8 servings*

Chocolate–Peanut Butter Pie

One lovely spring day when their crabapple tree was in full bloom and the lilacs were just coming out, I took one of these pies over to Vera and Aulden Wilsons' and we all sat at the kitchen table, along with their guest, Mrs. Emma Strong, and enjoyed it without even thinking that we were deprived because we were all, except for Mrs. Strong, on a diet.

Graham Cracker Crust (see p. 191)
2 cups 2% milk
1/4 cup chunky peanut butter
1 1.5-ounce package sugar-free Jell-O instant chocolate pudding
1 .9-ounce package Featherweight whipped sugar-free topping

Prepare graham cracker crust according to recipe and set aside. Place milk and peanut butter in mixer bowl and mix at medium speed until well blended, add pudding mix and mix at medium speed to blend well. As the pudding begins to thicken, pour it into the prepared pie crust and refrigerate until firm. Cut into 8 equal slices and serve 1 slice per serving, garnishing each piece with 2 Tablespoons whipped topping prepared according to directions on the package.

Nutritive values per serving: *cal 177, cho 17 gm, pro 5 gm, fat 10 gm, Na 352 mg*
Food exchanges per serving: *1 bread and 2 fat*
Low-sodium diets: *Use salt-free margarine when preparing the crust.*
Low-cholesterol diets: *Use skim milk instead of 2% milk, which will also cut the fat exchanges to 1 exchange. Do not use the whipped topping, which contains ingredients not suitable for a low-cholesterol diet.*
Yield: *1 9-inch pie, 8 servings*

Lemon Cream Pie

This lemon cream was my mother's special pie, which she made frequently. It can be made without the rind, but it is much better with grated rind and fresh lemon juice.

*Graham Cracker Crust (**see p. 191**)*
1/4 cup cornstarch
2 Tablespoons sugar
1/4 teaspoon salt
1/4 cup water at room temperature
1/4 cup lemon juice
3/4 cup (4 to 5 medium) eggs
2 cups boiling water
Grated rind from 1 lemon
Dry sugar substitute equal to 3/4 cup sugar
Diabetic whipped topping (optional)

Prepare crust according to recipe and set aside. Place cornstarch and sugar in mixer bowl and mix at medium speed to blend well. Add salt and 1/4 cup water and mix at medium speed until smooth. Add lemon juice and eggs and mix at medium speed until smooth. Add boiling water while mixing at low speed. Pour mixture into a small pan and cook and stir over medium heat until thickened and smooth. Remove from heat and add rind and sugar substitute. Cool about 5 minutes and then spread evenly in crust. Refrigerate until ready to serve and then divide into 8 equal pieces. Use 1 piece per serving, garnished with whipped topping if desired.

Nutritive values per serving: *cal 143, cho 15 gm, pro 4 gm, fat 8 gm, Na 196 mg*

Food exchanges per serving: *1 bread and 1 fat*

Low-sodium diets: *Omit salt. Use salt-free margarine when preparing the crust.*

Low-cholesterol diets: *Omit eggs. Use 3/4 cup liquid egg substitute. Omit whipped topping.*

Yield: *1 9-inch pie, 8 servings*

Raspberry Cloud Pie

Graham Cracker Crust (see p. 191)
2 cups fresh or frozen rhubarb cut into 1-inch pieces
1/4 cup water
cold water
1 .3-ounce package sugar-free raspberry gelatin
1 .9-ounce package Featherweight sugar-free whipped topping
fresh raspberries (optional)

Prepare graham cracker crust according to recipe and set aside. Cook rhubarb with 1/4 cup water in a small saucepan about 7 or 8 minutes or until very tender. Remove from heat and dissolve gelatin in the hot rhubarb. Add enough cold water to equal 1 1/2 cups of rhubarb mixture. Cool until syrupy. While the rhubarb mixture is cooling, prepare whipped topping as directed on the package. When the rhubarb mixture is cool and syrupy, stir into the whipped topping lightly so that it is streaked red and white. Spread the filling evenly in the pie crust and refrigerate until firm. Cut the pie into 6 equal pieces and garnish with a few fresh raspberries, if desired. Use 1 piece per serving.

Nutritive values per serving: *cal 122, cho 11 gm, pro 1 gm, fat 7 gm, Na 165 mg*

Food exchanges per serving: *2/3 bread and 1 fat*

Low-sodium diets: *Use salt-free margarine when preparing the crust.*

Low-cholesterol diets: *This recipe is not suitable because of ingredients in the topping.*

Yield: *1 9-inch pie, 6 servings*

Baked Cup Custard

1/2 cup (2 to 3 medium) eggs
2 cups skim milk
1 teaspoon vanilla
1/4 teaspoon salt
dry sugar substitute equal to 1/4 cup sugar
nutmeg (optional)
boiling water

Place eggs, milk, vanilla, salt and sugar substitute in a bowl and beat until well blended. Pour 1/4 of the custard into each of 4 custard cups. Sprinkle lightly with nutmeg and place all 4 of the cups in an 8-inch square cake pan. Pour boiling water about 1 1/2 inches deep around the cups and bake at 325°F for 1 hour or until a knife comes out clean from the center of the custard. Remove the custard from the hot water and cool to room temperature before refrigerating. Use 1 custard per serving.

Nutritive values per serving: *cal 91, cho 6 gm, pro 8 gm, fat 4 gm, Na 238 mg*
Food exchanges per serving: *1/2 skim milk and 1/2 medium-fat meat*
Low-sodium diets: *Omit salt.*
Low-cholesterol diets: *Substitute 1/2 cup liquid egg substitute for the eggs.*
Yield: *4 cup custards, 4 servings*

Fruit Fluff

The recipe was adapted from the Fruit Fluff recipes published in the magazine, *The Pleasures of Cooking,* with permission of the publisher, The Cuisinart Cooking Club. Dr. Crockett, who belongs to the club, suggested that this recipe, which was developed by their foods editor, Suzanne S. Jones, would be good for diabetic diets. It is a fabulous dessert, light and luscious when freshly made, and even better when it has been in the freezer a couple of hours. I also tested it using several stand mixers, and while you don't get results as good as those you get using the whip attachment of the Cuisinart food processor, it is still a marvelous dessert.

6 ounces frozen unsweetened strawberries (about 1 1/4 cups) or other fruits frozen without sugar
1 large egg white
1 1/2 teaspoons fresh or reconstituted lemon juice
1 Tablespoon sugar
6 1-gram packets Equal sugar substitute
1 1/2 teaspoons fruit liqueur or other spirits (optional)

With the metal blade of the food processor, finely chop the frozen fruit, scraping down the sides and top of the bowl as necessary. The fruit should look somewhat like powdered ice. (This step is very necessary and must be done in a food processor.)

Remove the metal blade from the Cuisinart food processor, lock the whisk adaptor to the motor shaft of the food processor and add the remaining ingredients. Connect the power unit to the adaptor with the whisks in place, pushing down as far as the unit will go.

Let the motor run until the mixture is light and fluffy and reaches the top of the beaters. Stop once to scrape the frozen fruit from the side of the work bowl. This will take from 3 to 5 minutes.

The fluff can be served immediately or spooned into parfait glasses or serving dishes and placed in the freezer for up to 2 hours. It can also be frozen solid, covered, for up to 2 days. If frozen solid, remove from the freezer 10 to 15 minutes before serving, to soften.

Notes

1. This may also be prepared in a stand mixer. Chop the food as directed in the food processor and then place it with the remaining ingredients in a stand mixer and mix, using a whip, at high speed for about 10 minutes. You should get 4 to 6 cups depending upon the stand mixer used. I got the best results with my Kitchen Aid mixer but I also got good results with several other good stand mixers.
2. An equal amount of other frozen unsweetened fruits may be substituted for the strawberries with no change in food exchanges.
3. The fruit-flavored liqueur enhances the fruit flavor but may be eliminated.
4. The fruit fluff may be garnished with a strawberry or other small bit of fresh or frozen fruit without changing the food exchange values.
5. One serving is 1/6 of the total amount of fluff which should be from 3/4 to 1 1/4 cups, depending upon the efficiency of your mixer.

Nutritive values per serving: *cal 27, cho 5 gm, pro 1 gm, fat negligible, Na 13 mg*

Food exchanges per serving: *1 vegetable*

Low-sodium diets: *May be used as written.*

Low-cholesterol diets: *May be used as written.*

Yield: *1 to 1 1/2 quarts, 6 servings*

Gelatin Trifle

Whenever I serve this, I remember how much Cracker and John Holton and their family liked it when we served it to them when they visited us in Chicago. They live in Clearwater, Florida, and I had forgotten that most southerners don't really serve the many, often elaborate gelatin desserts which we use here in the midwest. This one can be varied with different kinds of gelatins and fruits for the bottom layer but the vanilla pudding, banana and coconut should not be changed. (It looks beautiful in a glass bowl for a buffet or pot luck dinner.)

1.3-ounce package sugar-free strawberry gelatin dessert
2 cups boiling water
1 cup sliced unsweetened strawberries
1 1.1-ounce package sugar-free instant vanilla pudding
2 cups 2% milk
banana equal to 1 fruit exchange
1/4 cup shredded coconut

Dissolve gelatin in boiling water, cool to room temperature, add strawberries and pour into an 8- or 9-inch square pan or dish. Refrigerate until firm. Combine instant pudding and milk and mix thoroughly. Add sliced banana to pudding and pour over the gelatin. Sprinkle coconut evenly over the pudding and refrigerate until firm. Cut 3 × 3 for 9 equal squares. Use 1 square for each serving.

Nutritive values per serving: *cal 59, cho 8 gm, pro 2 gm, fat 2 gm, Na 209 mg*
Food exchanges per serving: *1/2 bread*
Low-sodium diets: *May be used as written.*
Low-cholesterol diets: *Use skim milk instead of 2% milk. Omit coconut and use banana equal to 2 fruit exchanges.*
Yield: *8- or 9-inch square trifle, 9 servings*

Pumpkin Pudding

Johnathan loves this, and so do Chuck and I. I can see why the Indians liked to eat cooked pumpkin with maple sugar and introduced it to our ancestors, who arrived in New England in the seventeenth century.

1 cup (5 to 6 medium) eggs
2 cups canned puréed pumpkin
1 15 1/2-ounce can evaporated skim milk
1/3 cup molasses
1/2 teaspoon salt
1 Tablespoon pumpkin pie spice
Sugar substitute equal to 1/2 cup sugar

Place eggs in mixer bowl and mix at low speed until thoroughly blended. Add pumpkin, evaporated milk, molasses, salt, spice and sugar substitute and mix at medium speed until well blended. Pour pudding into an 8-inch square baking pan and bake at 325°F about 1 hour or until a knife comes out clean from the center. Cut 3 × 4 into 12 equal portions and serve warm at room temperature or chilled with whipped topping using 1 square per serving.

Note: This pudding may also be used for pumpkin pie.

Nutritive values per serving: *cal 93, cho 12 gm, pro 6 gm, fat 3 gm, Na 156 mg. This recipe is a good source of fiber.*

Food exchanges per serving: *1 vegetable, 1/2 skim milk and 1/2 fat*

Low-sodium diets: *Omit salt.*

Low-cholesterol diets: *Omit eggs. Use 1 cup liquid egg substitute.*

Yield: *8-inch square pudding, 12 portions*

Rhubarb Cobbler

When I lived in Chicago, I missed having all of the fresh rhubarb I wanted, and now that we are out here in Iowa with a huge long row of rhubarb available, I use a great deal of it when it is in season and freeze even more because it is low in carbohydrate and high in fiber.

1 1/2 quarts (about 2 pounds) fresh or frozen rhubarb
1 3-ounce package regular strawberry flavored gelatin
2 Tablespoons cornstarch
dry sugar substitute equal to 1/2 cup sugar
1 cup rolled oats
3 Tablespoons melted margarine
1/2 teaspoon cinnamon
1/2 teaspoon Sweet 'n Low brown sugar substitute

Place rhubarb in a bowl. Combine strawberry gelatin, cornstarch and sugar substitute and mix well to blend. Pour the gelatin mixture over the rhubarb and toss the rhubarb in the mixture until all of the rhubarb pieces are coated. Place the rhubarb in an 8-inch square glass baking dish and sprinkle any remaining mixture over the rhubarb.

Stir the oatmeal, margarine, cinnamon and Sweet 'n Low together to mix well and then sprinkle evenly over the rhubarb. Bake at 350°F 40 to 45 minutes or until the rhubarb is soft and the topping is lightly browned. Cut the cobbler 3 × 3 to form 9 equal portions and use 1 portion per serving. Serve warm or cooled.

Nutritive values per serving: *cal 121, cho 18 gm, pro 2 gm, fat 5 gm, Na 45 mg. This recipe is a good source of fiber.*
Food exchanges per serving: *1 fruit and 1 fat*
Low-sodium diets: *May be used as written.*
Low-cholesterol diets: *May be used as written.*
Yield: *8-inch cobbler, 9 servings*

Rhubarb Pudding

Rhubarb isn't in season for very long, but we certainly take advantage of it when it is, and this is one of my favorite ways of using it.

1/2 cup (2 to 3 medium) eggs
1/3 cup sugar
2 teaspoons vanilla
1 cup all-purpose flour
1 Tablespoon baking powder
1/2 teaspoon salt
1 quart fresh rhubarb cut into 1-inch pieces
1/4 cup Sprinkle Sweet sugar substitute

Place eggs, sugar and vanilla in mixer bowl and mix at medium speed for 1/2 minute. Stir flour, baking powder and salt together to blend well, add to egg mixture and beat at medium speed only until blended together. Do not overbeat. Sprinkle rhubarb thoroughly with the sugar substitute and add to the batter, including any remaining sugar substitute. Mix well and spread evenly in an 8-inch square baking dish that has been well greased with margarine. Bake at 350°F for 30 to 35 minutes or until lightly browned and firm in the center. Cut 3 × 3 to yield 9 equal portions. Serve hot, using 1 portion per serving, with skim milk or Custard Sauce (see p. 206).

Nutritive values per serving: *cal 88, cho 15 gm, pro 3 gm, fat 2 gm, Na 249 mg. This recipe is a good source of fiber.*

Food exchanges per serving: *1 bread*

Low-sodium diets: *Omit salt. Use low sodium baking powder.*

Low-cholesterol diets: *Omit eggs. Use 1/2 cup liquid egg substitute.*

Yield: *9 servings*

Rice Pudding

3 cups boiling water
1/2 cup instant dry milk
1/3 cup long grain rice
1/2 cup (2 to 3 medium) eggs
1 Tablespoon cornstarch
2 teaspoons vanilla
1/2 teaspoon salt
12 1-gram packets Equal sugar substitute
cinnamon

Pour the water in the top of a double boiler over simmering hot water. Stir the milk into the hot water, add the rice and stir. Cook, stirring about every 5 or 10 minutes, for about 3/4 of an hour or until the rice is tender. Place the eggs in bowl and beat to blend well. Dissolve the cornstarch in the vanilla and add with the salt and sugar substitute to the eggs. Mix well. Beat 1 cup of the hot liquid from the rice into the egg mixture, then beat the egg mixture into the hot rice and cook over simmering water, stirring frequently, for another 5 minutes. Remove from stove and refrigerate until ready to serve, or serve warm, using 1/2 cup pudding per serving. Sprinkle with cinnamon before serving.

Nutritive values per serving: *cal 101, cho 14 gm, pro 5 gm, fat 2 gm, Na 222 mg*
Food exchanges per serving: *1 skim milk*
Low-sodium diets: *Omit salt.*
Low-cholesterol diets: *Omit eggs. Use 1/2 cup liquid egg substitute.*
Yield: *3 cups, 6 servings*

Strawberry Applesauce Gelatin

This recipe is so simple that I hesitate to include it in a recipe book, but it is so good that I wouldn't want you to miss it. I love it for dessert and I even put it on the table at breakfast and use it instead of jelly or jam on my bran muffins.

1 .3-ounce package sugar-free strawberry flavored gelatin
1 1/2 cups boiling water
1 cup unsweetened canned applesauce

Dissolve the gelatin in the boiling water, refrigerate until lukewarm and then add the applesauce. Pour into a dish and refrigerate until firm. Serve 1/2 cup (1/4 of the gelatin) per serving.

Nutritive values per serving: *cal 35, cho 7 gm, pro and fat negligible, Na 56 mg*
Food exchanges per serving: *1/2 fruit*
Low-sodium diets: *May be used as written.*
Low-cholesterol diets: *May be used as written.*
Yield: *about 2 cups, 4 servings*

Custard Sauce

Custard sauce is good over fruit, especially baked apples, puddings and gelatins. It can be served hot or cold and you can change the flavor by adding a little rum or other flavoring.

2 cups water
1/3 cup instant dry milk
1 1/2 Tablespoons cornstarch
1 egg
1 Tablespoon margarine
1 1/2 teaspoons vanilla
8 1-gram packets Equal sugar substitute

Combine water, dry milk and cornstarch together in top of a double boiler. Stir until smooth and then add egg. Beat with a rotary beater until smooth, add the margarine and place over simmering water. Cook, stirring frequently, until smooth and thickened and it coats a spoon. Remove from heat, add vanilla and serve hot or refrigerate until serving, using 1/4 cup per serving.

Nutritive values per serving: *cal 42, cho 4 gm, pro 2 gm, fat 2 gm, Na 39 mg*
Food exchanges per serving: *1 vegetable*
Low-sodium diets: *May be used as written.*
Low-cholesterol diets: *Omit egg. Use 1/4 cup liquid egg substitute.*
Yield: *2 cups, 8 servings*

INDEX

American Diabetes Association, Inc, 14
Applesauce cake, 165

Baked
  cup custard, 197
  halibut with paprika, 91
  meat balls, 74
  sandwiches, 75
Banana
  bran bread, 161
  cake, 170
Barley vegetable salad, 128
Basic fruit filling, 193
Bean soup, 58
Beans and beef, 77
Beef barley soup, 59
Black walnut cake, 167
Blueberry muffins, 153
Bouillon, 52
Braised beets and celery, 109
Bran cereals, 51
Bread flour, 137
Broccoli
  cauliflower salad, 127
  fritatta, 98
Brown gravy, 82
Buttercream frosting, 178
Buttermilk
  dry, 50
  walnut muffins, 152
Butternut squash casserole, 116

Cajun style catfish, 92
Cake mix formula, 162
Caramel rolls, 148
Cassata, 170
Cheese sauce, 101
Chef's french dressing, 133
Cherry cheese cake, 172
Chicken
  gravy, 90
  lasagna, 84
  potato salad, 122
Chili with turkey, 87
Chinese spinach, 114
Chocolate
  almond cake, 177
  cake, 168
  chip rolls, 148
  oat bran cookies with chocolate chips, 184
  peanut butter pie, 194
  sauce, 179
  topped cake, 177
Cinnamon rolls, 146
Coconut
  chocolate chip cookies, 185
  oatmeal cookies, 186
Coleslaw, 129
Combination foods exchange list, 38–39
Complex carbohydrates, 18
Corn soup, 62
Country style tomatoes, 117
Cranberry muffins, 153
Cream
  sauces, 101–2
  of vegetable soup, 61
Creamed
  cauliflower, 108
  salmon and peas, 93
  spinach with peanuts, 114
Creole summer squash, 115
Custard sauce, 206

Date bran cake, 173
Diabetic salad dressing, 134
Dipper sizes, 150
DITN (*Diabetes in the News*), 15
Double chocolate cookies, 182
Dundee cake, 174

Egg bread, 139
Escalloped asparagus and eggs, 99
Exchange use form, 43

Fast rising yeast, 137
Fat exchanges list, 35–37
Fiber
  crude, 16
  dietary, 16
  types, 17
  water soluble, 20
Food exchange values, 23
Free foods list, 37–38
Fruit
  exchanges list, 32–34
  fluff, 198

Gelatin trifle, 200
Gênoise, 176
Graham
  bread, 142
  cracker crust, 191
Greens, preparation, 120–21

Hamburger with brown rice, 78

Legumes, 106
Lemon
  applesauce salad, 125
  cream pie, 195
Light bran bread, 140
Liquid egg substitute, 47
Low calorie foods, 46
Low sodium foods, 47

Macaroni
  and cheese, 100
  slaw, 130
Margarine, 52
Meal patterns, 44
Meat
  balls,74
  exchanges list, 27–31
Milk
  exchanges list, 34–35
  instant dry, 50
Minestrone soup, 62
Mushroom tomato soup, 64

Oat bran
  cereal, 20
  muffins, 154
  pie crust, 192
  Vera's cookies, 188
Occasional foods exchange list, 39–40

Pan sizes, 164
Pasticchio, 79
Pecan bran muffins, 155
Pineapple
  apple and celery salad, 126
  bran muffins, 156
  chicken, 86
Poached fish, 94
Polka dot coffee cake, 159
Pot roasted turkey legs, 88
Potato soup, 65
Pumpkin pudding, 201

Raisin
  bran bread, 143
  bran quick bread, 158
  spice cookies, 187
Raspberry cloud pie, 196
Recipe analysis, 68, 76
Rhubarb
  cobbler, 202
  muffins, 153
  pudding, 203
Rice pudding, 204
Rye bread, 145

Salmon
  loaf, 95
  luncheon salad, 123
Salt-free broth, 55
Sample menu patterns, 45
Saucy beans and mushrooms, 109
Sauerkraut with applesauce, 113
Scalloped cabbage, 111
Shredded carrots, 107
Soup categories, 54
Southern-style greens, 112
Spiced peach salad, 126
Starch/bread exchanges list, 24
Steamed vegetables, 105
Stewed tomatoes, 118
Stir-fried pork and vegetables, 83
Strawberry applesauce gelatin, 205
Sugar, 48
Sugar substitutes, 48–50
Sweet
  cabbage salad, 131
  sour cabbage, 111

Tartar sauce, 97
Tomato meat sauce for spaghetti, 80
Tunafish
  macaroni and broccoli, 96
  mold, 124
Turkey loaf, 89

Vegetable
  exchanges list, 31–32
  oil, 51
  parfait, 132
Vera's oat bran cookies, 188
Vinegar and oil dressing, 135

Yeast, 51